Living
Professionalism

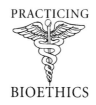

PRACTICING

BIOETHICS

Practicing Bioethics
General Editor: Mark G. Kuczewski, Ph.D.
Neiswanger Institute for Bioethics and Health Policy
Loyola University Chicago

The Practicing Bioethics series provides readers with insight into the professional practices by which bioethicists, physicians, nurses, and other healthcare practitioners address current ethical issues. These works cut through the usual back-and-forth of abstract arguments to examine how to resolve dilemmas in the clinic, at the bedside, and in the boardroom. Volumes address practical issues such as professionalism in healthcare, clinical bioethics consultation, death and dying, and clinical genetics. These books provide a distinctive resource for educating practitioners-in-training such as medical students and residents, allied health professionals, healthcare administrators, and policymakers, as well as students of bioethics at the graduate and undergraduate level.

Editorial Advisory Board

Mark Aulisio, Ph.D., Case Western Reserve University
Rebecca Dresser, J.D., Washington University School of Law
Kevin FitzGerald, S.J., Ph.D., Georgetown University Medical Center
Joel Frader, M.D., Northwestern University, Feinberg School of Medicine
Leslie Francis, J.D., Ph.D., University of Utah
Susan Dorr Goold, M.D., M.H.S.A., M.A., University of Michigan Medical School
D. Micah Hester, Ph.D., University of Arkansas for Medical Sciences
Alex London, Ph.D., Carnegie Mellon University
Laurel Lyckholm, M.D., Virginia Commonwealth University School of Medicine
M. Therese Lysaught, Ph.D., University of Dayton
Kathryn Montgomery, Ph.D., Northwestern University, Feinberg School of Medicine
Daniel Sulmasy, O.F.M., M.D., Ph.D., New York Medical College
Griffin Trotter, M.D., Ph.D., Center for Health Care Ethics, St. Louis University
Delese Wear, Ph.D., Northeastern Ohio Universities College of Medicine
Gladys White, R.N., Ph.D., American Nurses Association

Titles in the Series

Living Professionalism

Reflections on the Practice of Medicine

Edited by Erin A. Egan
and Patricia M. Surdyk

ROWMAN & LITTLEFIELD PUBLISHERS, INC.
Lanham • Boulder • New York • Toronto • Plymouth, UK

Samford University Library

ROWMAN & LITTLEFIELD PUBLISHERS, INC.

Published in the United States of America
by Rowman & Littlefield Publishers, Inc.
A wholly owned subsidiary of The Rowman & Littlefield Publishing Group, Inc.
4501 Forbes Boulevard, Suite 200, Lanham, Maryland 20706
www.rowmanlittlefield.com

Estover Road
Plymouth PL6 7PY
United Kingdom

Copyright © 2006 by Rowman & Littlefield Publishers, Inc.

All rights reserved. No part of this publication may be reproduced,
stored in a retrieval system, or transmitted in any form or by any
means, electronic, mechanical, photocopying, recording, or otherwise,
without the prior permission of the publisher.

British Library Cataloguing in Publication Information Available

Library of Congress Cataloging-in-Publication Data

Living professionalism : reflections on the practice of medicine / edited
    by Erin A. Egan and Patricia M. Surdyk.
    p. ; cm. — (Practicing bioethics)
    Includes bibliographical references and index.
    ISBN-13: 978-0-7425-4851-0 (pbk. : alk. paper)
    ISBN-10: 0-7425-4851-1 (pbk. : alk. paper)
    1. Medical ethics. 2. Physicians—Professional ethics. 3. Clinical
    competence.   I. Egan, Erin A., 1970–   II. Surdyk, Patricia M., 1947–   .
III. Series.
    [DNLM: 1. Medicine. 2. Professional Practice. 3. Professional Auto-
nomy.   W 21 L785 2006]
    R725.5.L58 2006
    610—dc22   2006009439

Printed in the United States of America

⊗™ The paper used in this publication meets the minimum requirements of
American National Standard for Information Sciences—Permanence of Paper for
Printed Library Materials, ANSI/NISO Z39.48-1992.

R
725.5
.L58
2006

Table of Contents

Acknowledgments

We extend sincere thanks to:

- David C. Leach, M.D., executive director of the Accreditation Council for Graduate Medical Education (ACGME), whose challenge to collect stories on professionalism resulted in this effort.
- Mark Kuczewski, Ph.D., director of the Neiswanger Institute for Bioethics and Health Policy as well as senior editor of the Practicing Bioethics series, whose support of this project from the outset and unflagging patience provided the encouragement we needed to continue.
- Gwen L. Nichols, M.D., Norma E. Wagoner, Ph.D., and Alison S. Clay, M.D., whose scholarly reflections are grounded in their personal commitment to living the professional values about which they write with such skill.

And finally,

- Those individuals whose stories and reflections provide evidence of the understanding and lived experience of professionalism we hope to facilitate in the ongoing development of all who use this volume.

Erin A. Egan, M.D, J.D.
Patricia M. Surdyk, Ph.D.

1

Living Professionalism in Medicine: An Introduction

Patricia M. Surdyk, Ph.D., editor

"LOOKING" FOR PROFESSIONALISM

"**Y**ou know it when you see it" has become an almost proverbial response to the question, "What is professionalism in medicine?" If you are a clerkship director or residency program director, you might respond this way as you attempt to define, foster, and assess specific values associated with professionalism in trainees. If you are a medical student or resident, you might find yourself responding similarly when you are asked to judge the professionalism of your peers or mentors or when your patients are asked to judge your behavior. If you have the unforgettable experience of observing a colleague who demonstrates extraordinary professionalism in a particular situation, you are certain you have witnessed professional values in action. Sadly, the opposite can also be true; you know precisely and painfully when professionalism is missing.

Although concerns about professionalism in medicine are not new, the most recent attention it has received arises in part from what can be seen as an erosion of public trust in the professions as a whole (Surdyk, Lynch, and Leach 2003). These concerns underscore the need for a better understanding of professionalism and for demonstrated evidence of how the values that give meaning to the medical profession are applied in practice. In response to not only these concerns, but also in support of improved education through outcomes assessment, expectations of accrediting and certifying bodies, i.e., the Liaison Committee on Medical Education (LCME 2005), the Accreditation Council for Graduate Medical Education (ACGME 1999), and the American Board of Medical Specialties (ABMS 1999) have added to the concerted effort to teach and assess professionalism. These organizations include professionalism as one of the competencies that medical students, residents, and practicing physicians are expected to demonstrate. Values associated with professionalism are expected to be taught and modeled; these values should be apparent in interactions with patients, with each other, with other health professionals, and with society.

Over the past decade, a growing body of medical literature has provided a means to address the ambiguity surrounding professionalism. This literature has helped to identify those characteristics that define professionalism (Arnold 2002), best methods to teach and communicate professional values (ACGME 2004), and approaches to assessing whether these efforts have been successful (Gordon 2003; Papadakis, Loeser, and Healy 2001). These resources have helped create a deeper understanding of the contract medicine has with society (Cruess and Cruess 1999). They have shown us how professionalism is a dynamic characteristic rather than a constant state, a lifelong experience of resolving conflicts in context (Ginsburg et al. 2002), motivated by values such as honor and integrity. Regrettably, they have also provided evidence that a lack of professionalism and associated communication skills frequently result in serious breaches of medical conduct (Hickson 2002).

Efforts to teach and assess professionalism, however, are not about creating doctor-saints. They are meant to support one's ability to rise above self-interest when confronted by the mysteries of life and death or when simply trying to deal with a particularly difficult patient. Learning about professionalism reveals the commitment required of those who practice medicine and expected by those for whom they provide care.

LIVING PROFESSIONALISM

This book focuses on living the values of professionalism in medicine. It is a collection of stories and reflections, the intent of which is simply to share real-life experiences of professionalism. "We know it when we see it" is true. It follows, therefore, that we must first define professional values for ourselves in order to identify how, in turn, to act professionally.

To put it a slightly different way, after reflecting on—not merely reading through—the contributed essays in this volume, a variation of the response to "What is professionalism?" might be along the lines of "I know it as I learn to live it." Such a variation differentiates this book within the body of the literature on professionalism described above. These essays do not provide information to be digested; the book is not a research project. The personal contributions are not meant to provide new and improved means of meeting accreditation or certification requirements. They provide no definitive answers for questions that defy simplistic responses. The contents are designed for medical students, residents, and those responsible for their formation. These essays are meant for personal reflection and above all for thoughtful discussion with mentors, with peers, with others throughout the health care provider community who care about acting professionally.

A TOOL TO FACILITATE REFLECTION

Separate types of contributed works are contained in this volume. It opens with invited essays by thoughtful leaders in their respective areas of medicine and medical education, who provide personal guidance and scholarly direction in thinking through particular issues related to professionalism. Stories and essays submitted in response to an open invitation make up the second type of contribution. The request for these works was sent to various organizations, disseminated in person to interested individuals, and posted on the website of the Neiswanger Institute for Bioethics and Health Policy (at which one of the editors is a faculty member) in early 2005. The request was to present stories or cases from personal experience in response to the questions, "What is professionalism?" and "How is it learned?" The contributions were to enhance the understanding of professionalism in medicine by identifying professional behaviors in practice, supporting the ongoing development of professionalism education in medicine, and publishing original, reflective work about professionalism.

But why choose to tell stories, to write reflections, in the first place? "Good doctoring" and "becoming a physician" classes/experiences in medical school or expectations of developing reflective portfolios in residency are often viewed by students and residents as "busy work," taking precious time away from practicing medicine. In the first of the two invited essays, "The Power of Narrative Reflections," Gwen L. Nichols, M.D., reminds us that narrative is at the heart of the doctor-patient relationship. Physicians always have stories to tell. Dr. Nichols shows how reflective narrative used in the manner of the contributions to this book and through other various applications is one effective means of achieving the authenticity required to live professionalism.

The second invited essay, "Generational Differences and the Challenges to Achieving a More Reflective Definition for Professionalism," addresses the "elephant in the room": How do different generations of doctors speak to each other about professional values which often appear in opposition? Generational differences are seldom overlooked and frequently present, but they are hardly ever addressed with such honesty, forthrightness, and conscientious attention to underlying causes as here by Norma Wagoner, Ph.D., and Alison Clay, M.D.

The personal responses to the open request for submissions that make up the second type of contributed work seemed to align themselves naturally around several themes: how medical students and residents learn the values associated with professionalism, how medical educators seek to foster professionalism directly through various organized learning activities, and how attempts to live professional values frequently result in personal conflict or, as the case may be, in the opportunity to resolve conflict, unbeknownst to the individual acting on his or her values. The final contribution is that of a patient who summarizes those characteristics he views as most important to physicians' professionalism.

JUST "DO" IT

There are lessons to be learned about professionalism. As one contributor states, "My heritage of medicine does not endow me with an unlearned ability to speak [the] language[s] of professionalism. Opportunities to learn [this language] must be recognized and embraced" (see Boyte, p. 53–54). Using narrative to share stories, exploring the meaning of actions, and meeting head-on the differences that seemingly divide the generations are the means we have chosen to aid such learning. This book offers no easy answers. We hope instead that the efforts of the individuals who willingly shared their experiences for this work will provide material for reflection, for interaction, and, most importantly, for living out the values of professionalism with passion and commitment.

Why learn about professionalism when, indeed, it appears difficult to define and challenging to live? Perhaps the poet Rilke provides the best answer to spending one's life in service of patients: "Have patience with everything unresolved in your heart and to try to love the questions themselves. . . . And the point is to live everything. Live the questions now. Perhaps then, someday far in the future, you will gradually, without even noticing it, live your way into the answer" (Rilke 1993).

REFERENCES

Accreditation Council for Graduate Medical Education (ACGME). 1999. The ACGME Outcome Project: General Competencies [cited 18 November 2005]. Available from www.acgme.org/outcome/comp/compFull.asp.

———. 2004. *Advancing Education in Medical Professionalism* [cited 10 October 2005]. Available from: www.acgme.org/outcome/implement/Profm_resource.pdf.

American Board of Medical Specialties (ABMS). 1999. Description of the Competent Physician [cited 18 November 2005]. Available from www.abms.org/Downloads/Publications/3Approved%20Initiatives%20for%20MOC.pdf.

Arnold, L. 2002. Assessing professional behavior: yesterday, today, and tomorrow. *Academic Medicine* 77(6): 516–22.

Cruess, R., and S. Cruess. 1999. Renewing professionalism: an opportunity for medicine. *Academic Medicine* 74(8): 878–84.

Ginsburg, S., et al. 2002. The anatomy of the professional lapse: bridging the gap between traditional frameworks and students' perceptions. *Academic Medicine* 77(6): 516–22.

Gordon, J. 2003. Assessing students' personal and professional portfolios and interviews. *Medical Education* 37(4): 335–40.

Hickson, G., et al. 2002. Patient complaints and malpractice risk. *Journal of the American Medical Association* 287(22): 2951–57.

Liaison Committee on Medical Education (LCME). 2005. *Structure and Functions of Medical School, ED-1-Al.* Washington, D.C.: Association of American Medical Colleges [cited 18 November 2005]. Available from www.lcme.org/functions2005oct.pdf.

Papadakis, M., H. Loeser, and K. Healy. 2001. Early detection and evaluation of professionalism deficiencies in medical students: one school's approach. *Academic Medicine* 76(11): 1100–1106.

Rilke, R. M. 1993. *Letters to a Young Poet.* Translated by M. D. Norton. New York: W.W. Norton & Company.

Surdyk, P., D. Lynch, and D. Leach. 2003. Professionalism: identifying current themes. *Current Opinion in Anesthesiology* 16: 597–602.

2

The Power of Narrative Reflections

Gwen L. Nichols, M.D.

NARRATIVE, PROFESSIONALISM, AND
THE DOCTOR-PATIENT RELATIONSHIP

Professionalism can be described as a code of conduct agreed upon by colleagues, patients, and society in general. Major elements of medical professionalism include placing patients' interests first, acquiring and maintaining skills essential for practice, and displaying qualities of humanism including empathy and compassion. As described by the American Board of Internal Medicine's "Project Professionalism" (ABIM 1999), the most important elements of professionalism are altruism, accountability, duty, excellence, honor and integrity, and respect for others. At first glance, these precepts seem straightforward, but the expectations of personal sacrifice and lifelong commitment to placing the needs of others before one's own are not so simple. Unwavering, long-term empathy and altruism take an emotional toll on physicians. Medical professionalism calls for a commitment that professionals in other fields are not uniformly required to make. So how do we encourage and reward altruism, empathy, excellence, and integrity in the demanding world of modern medicine?

Empathy is the ability to imagine oneself in another's place and to be able to comprehend the ideas, feelings, and wishes of another person. To be empathic, therefore, requires a number of important elements. First is self-awareness—how you react to the emotionally powered situations common in the practice of medicine. Second is awareness of others—the ability to listen and attend to the feelings, factual content, and emotional content of what another person is saying to you. Third, imagination is critical for empathy. Imagination allows you to place yourself theoretically in the situation of another, allowing you to place the other person's reactions in context. As a physician-teacher, I am acutely aware that the great majority of students entering medical school are enthusiastic, hopeful, and altruistic, having a true desire to help others. Yet time and again I hear stories of physicians who are impersonal, technology-driven, and frankly depressed, characteristics in clear conflict with professional ideals. The practice of medicine has changed dramatically over the past several decades, and with the change has come a loss of physician autonomy, an increase in technology, increased patient expectations, and a decrease in available time to spend with patients. Patients complain bitterly of the loss of personal interaction with physicians, the loss of the "human touch," the loss of a meaningful physician-patient relationship. Public perception, both through personal accounts and in the media, corroborate the impersonal nature of many interactions in our current health care system. Not only patients, but many physicians mourn the loss of the personal interactions in medicine. The exceptional relationships physicians are allowed to have with patients are what first brought many physicians to the practice of medicine. What in the process of professional education can we do to reverse this trend and help physicians avoid becoming distanced, insensitive, and uncaring? One method to fight dehumanization of medicine is to be more aware of the stories or narratives we hear in the day-to-day process of being a physician.

The stereotype of the impersonal physician exists in stark contrast to the humanity, caring, kindness, bravery, and sacrifice I see daily in physicians working in the hospital. But I cannot ignore that I also see physicians who display the opposite. When asked what makes a good doctor, I often reply "common sense." While this seems a blithe avoidance of the question, some of the simplest tasks of listening and thinking may be the first place to start in maintaining professionalism. In the patient's mind, the sensitivity of the physician, his or her use of the right words, can mean as much as scientific brilliance. This approach is counterintuitive to the way medicine is taught, which is often at the expense of common sense. From the preclinical years, with hours of technical lectures and constant examinations, to the clinical years and residency, where lack of sleep, food, and attention to bodily needs are commonplace, much of medical training promotes the antithesis of common sense. In fact, medical training often, by design, strips the physician-trainee of self-awareness, forcing him or her to rely more on intellect and "facts" than on feelings. From their earliest experiences in anatomy, the focus for trainees is on professional distance, detachment, and attitudes that favor mental processes. Physical and emotional responses are for patients. The more we physicians see ourselves as "different," the further we move from comprehending the patients' needs, and, therefore, the further we distance ourselves from promoting patient satisfaction with medical care. Narrative reflection, writing, and attending to our patients' stories can help us find more professional satisfaction for ourselves and for our patients.

Among many perspectives through which it might be viewed, the doctor-patient relationship might be considered as a series of narratives. The stories patients tell us are not important only to the patient or only to record a patient's history on a chart. The relationships we have with our patients as we hear their stories have a great impact on our sense of satisfaction, personal worth, and ability to practice the high professional standards we take an oath to maintain. One method of maintaining professional integrity is to honor and reflect on the amazing intimate human stories we as physicians are privileged to hear. These personal narratives are unique to medical practice. How we act and react based upon these stories plays a substantial role in our interactions with patients, our interactions with our peers, and our role in society.

WHY PAY ATTENTION TO NARRATIVE?

There are two reasons for attending to and recalling the stories we hear as well as the stories we ourselves have to share. The first is that by realizing that patients' histories are stories and narrative, we become better listeners, more able to get to the essence of patients' histories, their needs, and, eventually, their illness and health. A critical part of being a medical professional is our ability to interpret these stories, to place them in a context of medical facts, and to react both competently and empathically to these stories in order to help the patient. The second reason to reflect upon patients' stories is as a way of unburdening ourselves from the human sorrows and tragedies we see in our practice and of remembering the joys, successes, and amazing human spirit we witness as physicians. Telling our own stories, our deep reactions to our patients and to our lives as physicians, strengthens our resolve and allows us to continue to practice medicine as a profession rather than just as a job. Reflection allows us to avoid rushing through the very human part of being a doctor. So there exists both the story of the medical history as told by our patients and the stories we tell in relating that history. While in the medical chart and on medical rounds it is appropriate to detail medical facts, the history we hear is not just facts, as patients are not just their vital signs. Neither are we, as physicians, merely automatons who record and recite medical facts. How do we relate to these stories, the parts not suitable for the medical chart, in an appropriate fashion? Some physicians have chosen medical writing (novels, lay articles, creative writing for medical journals). Clearly, this is not the route for every physician. Nonetheless, we are storytellers (Verghese 2001) by virtue of being part of each patient's story through our interactions with patients and our writing about them in the medical chart. How can we expand the use of narrative to maintain professionalism?

Let us start with narrative as it pertains to listening and detailing the patient's history in the process of providing care. What we may take away from medical training is that the subjective, the personal, and the emotional should not be included in what we relate about patients. We are taught that decisions should be made solely in the context of medical facts, and our writing should follow a format that is standardized. We shun idiosyncrasy. We look for commonalities. We strive for standardization, certainty, and reproducibility. We look for common threads that pull divergent stories together into a coherent diagnosis. Writing in the medical chart is intended to exclude the personal voice. Medical notes are written in a prescribed format that may focus on the patient's reactions, but not the physician's reaction. What is not emphasized is that the history is a patient's story and is subject to both the patient's and the doctor's interpretation of historical "facts." Relating that story has emotional content and context. Although placing these thoughts in the medical chart is proscribed, these elements of the patients' stories nonetheless affect us. They can haunt us, make us angry, make us suspicious, make us smile. Recognizing cases as "stories" is the point of narrative medicine. Recognizing and making a place for the emotional content of these stories (which is not in the formal medical chart) and having a way to describe the many thoughts and emotions these stories invoke, is the essential nature of narrative medicine. It is not a great literary construct, meant only for those who write medical novels or study classical literature in the context of medicine. Rather it is a way to examine the stories of our patients in the context of our own stories, to recognize our own emotional reactions, and to help us understand our patients and ourselves as human beings. It is in this context that the interactions with our patients make being a physician difficult, draining, dramatic, and fulfilling (Horowitz et al. 2003).

NARRATIVE COMPETENCE AND NARRATIVE MEDICINE

Narrative competence has been defined as the ability and the skills necessary to recognize, interpret, and respond both medically and empathically to the stories our patients relate to us (Kleinman 1988; Charon 2001a). My colleague Rita Charon, M.D., has coined the term "narrative medicine" to describe the process practiced by physicians of using medical narrative for giving a framework to medical reasoning, the doctor-patient relationship, empathy, ethics, and professionalism (Charon 2001b). Dr. Charon describes narrative medicine as the acquisition of skills in recognizing singularities about people or events, adopting another's perspective, decoding complex oral and written texts, tolerating ambiguity and uncertainty, and honoring stories of self and other (Charon 2004). The ability to entertain multiple perspectives, creativity/imagination, and skills of emotional accessibility in the face of those who are different are not straightforward skills to learn or maintain, particularly when working under time and technical pressures. Through new efforts to provide health professionals the opportunity to gain narrative skills, as well as the time and opportunity for reflection, it is hoped that physicians will have an increased capacity to listen, diagnose accurately, and develop therapeutic relationships with patients.

Understanding the patient's story is and has always been an integral and inherent art of the practice of medicine. The emerging change is that we recognize now with greater clarity the role of narrative in professional development. Medical schools and residency programs are more frequently encouraging trainees to write about or speak about clinical experiences (Brady, Corbie-Smith, and Branch 2002; Branch et al. 1993; Coulehan 1995; Hatem and Ferrara 2001; Marshall and O'Keefe 1995; Poirier, Ahrens, and Brauner 1998). More trainees and professionals are offered opportunities for reflective writing. First-year medical students may write about their feelings in dissecting the human body. Preclinical students in courses on the doctor-patient relationship may write about patients' lives. Medical students are encouraged to write fiction, poetry, or letters from imaginary patients to foster sensitivity and humane care. Physicians write about the meaningful experiences in their practice to process the emotional fallout from these clinical experiences. This process of writing and reflection may be formalized or individualized, but it is increasingly recognized as having an important place in medical training. Some of the programs include reading the published narratives of physician/writers (Wear and Nixon 2002). The poems and essays written by others with similar experiences provide an excellent starting point to reflect on and discuss the personal and professional challenges common to physicians.

APPLICATION OF NARRATIVE MEDICINE

The Program in Narrative Medicine at Columbia University has promoted, in the third and fourth years of study, the use of what has been termed parallel charts (DasGupta and Charon 2004). Students are asked, in addition to maintaining traditional records on their patients' progress, to track the emotions they and their patients experience while in the hospital. Once a week, they meet to read their accounts to each other, and they have found that recalling these memories, sorrows, and successes, the many feelings that accompany patient care, can influence the care they give, now and in the future. In a recent study (Rita Charon, personal communication), the parallel chart method was rated by 82 percent of the participating students as beneficial, both as a therapeutic outlet for the emotional trials of medical school and residency and as a more effective preparation for conversations with patients and their families. Faculty members concurred that students involved with the program were better equipped to perform both intake interviewing and evaluation of patients' needs than nonparticipating peers. Bearing witness to and receiving feedback about the natural empathic human emotions that occur in caring for the ill validate these experiences and allow students and physicians not to feel alone in their sensitivity and thoughtfulness. Such activities are not meant to function as support groups or counseling sessions. Rather, narrative training seeks to be an integral part of professional development and maintenance of professional integrity throughout a physician's career. Rather than "medicalizing" sensitivity and empathy, the parallel chart, narrative writing, and narrative reading with discussion encourages the view that interpreting and expressing the emotional content of patients' stories is normal and beneficial to remaining a sensitive and caring professional. If "gallows humor" has a place in medicine, surely reflecting on the more empathetic stories of our patients and our colleagues should be at the heart of practice.

The emerging programs using narrative in health care settings thus allow professionals to share a common perspective. Writing about and discussing our experiences as physicians provides an avenue toward professionalism: consciousness, responsibility, ethicality, diagnostic reasoning, and alliance building with patients.

OBSTACLES TO RECOGNIZING THE IMPORTANCE OF NARRATIVE IN MEDICAL EDUCATION

But why isn't hearing and relating the patient's story a "natural" part of medical practice? An obvious answer is the change in our history taking. One of the dramatic forces leading away from the best medical history taking and listening to patients' stories is the necessity of "compliance," i.e., the performance and documentation of particular elements in history taking for reimbursement. The physician is now required to document and ascertain a set list of required elements in order to be paid for the patient visit. While ostensibly a mechanism to assure not only that the work is being done but also to confirm the thoroughness of the approach, history taking often leads us to create a laundry-list review of systems. We pose questions in rapid-fire succession instead of listening and allowing the conversation to take us closer to the patient's concerns. This process occurs in an increasingly shorter time frame. Clearly, these circumstances become a recipe for poor history taking and poor listening. The more we direct the patient's history, the further we move away from a "patient-centered" history (Platt et al. 2001; Benbassat and Baumal 2004) toward a "reimbursement-worthy" history. The idea of a thorough review of systems makes good sense. Nevertheless, focusing on a piece of paper and marking off all the boxes in a prescribed order keeps us from focusing on the patient. Patients sense this, too. Doctors are often more intent upon asking "their" questions than on hearing the patient's answers. To quote William Osler: "If you have enough time, the patient will tell you everything you need to know about their illness." Unfortunately, rigid use of preformatted questionnaires moves us further away from letting the patient tell us what we need to know.

Evidence-based medicine and "decision tree" analysis have also affected our response to hearing the patient's story. We run the risk of being more concerned with making the pieces of the puzzle fit instead of leaving our minds open enough to hear what the patient is telling us. Striving for efficiency in the medical history, in the exam, and in the office is becoming a fact of modern medical practice. But while reproducible, empirically valid, and scientifically designed study of our treatments and their efficacy move the profession forward, the most beneficial medical history may not be as easily structured. Doctors must interpret signs and symptoms in the context of what the patient's story and physical findings suggest, and a less thorough story or a poorly obtained or poorly interpreted story following only a directed course of set elements stifles the ability to discover critical elements of the history. We all use selective hearing. "Red flags" abound; we naturally tune into important information and we tend to tune out other parts of conversations. We cannot deny that our emotional impressions color our clinical impressions. We apply our diagnoses and therapeutic suggestions in the context of the patient's history and individual traits, wishes, and goals. Patients rarely conform to the decision tree.

The scientific mind-set we acquire through the medical school curriculum prepares us well for finding the key elements of the history and delivering a diagnosis based on key facts. We search in the history for elements confirming our clinical suspicions—a reductionist approach with an empiric basis. We then proceed with tests to confirm our suspicions. What we fail to do as successfully is to study what role our interpretive skills play in "hearing" key elements of the history. If we do not convey empathy, if we do not listen well, we may not be given the key elements of the history to interpret. Citing these concerns is in no way a call to eliminate empiric reasoning. Rather it is a call to validate the use of the patient's story to help us get to the real history. It is recognition of the fact that when we converse with others, we do not simply analyze the content of the conversation; we also react to the context.

How does the patient behave? Angry, frustrated, pained, fatigued? What words are used to describe the pain? Is there exaggeration, minimalization? What feelings does the patient evoke in us? All these factors play a role in our impression of the medical facts and may alter our impression of what the patient's problem may be, given the facts and the interpretive paradigm we employ.

One limitation of traditional medical education curricula that focus on the doctor-patient relationship or professionalism is that these programs are offered as "special" courses, separate from the core curriculum (Bardes 2004). These topics, therefore, tend to be undervalued or are thought to be "soft," nonscientific, and therefore less important to becoming a professional. Recognizing that these "special" attributes are critical not only in medical school but also for practicing professionals may be the first step toward effectively addressing the terrible dissatisfaction with patient-physician interactions one may otherwise experience in professional practice.

CAN NARRATIVE HAVE A ROLE IN A PHYSICIAN'S PRACTICE?

We have discussed how paying attention to patient narratives and narrative competence may help us understand our patients, and we have mentioned a few of the programs available. So how do we continue narrative competence after medical school and how does it benefit physicians? The narrative oncology program developed at Columbia arose as a consequence of a number of emotionally and ethically charged clinical situations on the oncology unit and our recognition that we had no effective way to discuss the emotions the staff members were experiencing in the course of caring for cancer patients. We realized that "counseling" would make these emotions seem as if they were a problem to correct and not a normal experience, so we sought a way to gain acceptance for discussions of painful and difficult topics. Writing as a way to introduce sensitive topics became an excellent way to begin necessary discussions. Our groups included nurses, social workers, and junior and senior physicians meeting every two weeks, writing about a patient or a patient-related experience while protecting patient identifiers. The results of this project were as anticipated. Participants found a sense of support, a sharing of sadness, and a feeling of community.

Unanticipated results were that the group gained a better understanding of where roles of different professionals may conflict. As a result, team building occurred, as did increased sensitivity to colleagues from different disciplines. Many participants were surprised at the level of heartfelt emotions in the disciplines other than their own and how little time we spend with our colleagues in nursing and social work discussing nonmedical issues. The most surprising result from our program in narrative oncology was the development of constructive changes for improving clinical care that were a direct result of sharing these narratives. In the end, the narrative interventions had ongoing, tangible benefits for our patients. Even after the trial period was completed, a large group continued the sessions as a way to "decompress" and brainstorm on difficult patients and difficult emotions. Few of the participants considered themselves writers or diarists prior to this exercise, but the intensity of the writing was nonetheless uniformly poignant and always led to fruitful discussions.

Why else should hospitals allocate resources to encourage writing for caregivers? One answer is to stop the great loss of trained professionals to what has been described as "burnout" (Maslach, Schaufeli, and Leiter 2001). Burnout is a response to chronic emotional stressors on the job and is defined by exhaustion, cynicism, and inefficacy in the workplace. All these characteristics are the antithesis of professionalism. Research has found some identifiable job characteristics that predispose the development of burnout in human services, including provision of demanding care, a high number of patients who are ill, prevalence of negative feedback or outcomes, and a scarcity of resources and support services. Current medical practice fits these criteria quite well. In an effort at self-protection, caregivers may create emotional distance or detachment, which can interfere with job functioning. Burnout has been associated with negative organizational outcomes related to changes in job performance, including absenteeism, intention to leave the job, increased personal conflict, and lower effectiveness. It may also lead to serious personal health consequences, including depression and substance abuse. These findings have direct consequences on the quality of patient care; a number of studies have found a direct relationship between medical staff turnover and risk-adjusted mortality scores, severity-adjusted length of stay, and medical errors (Maslach, Schaufeli, and Leiter 2001).

In a study of physicians in my specialty, oncology, a remarkable 85 percent of respondents said career-related burnout was affecting their personal and social lives. A similar questionnaire-based study in cancer clinicians found that 28 percent experienced psychiatric disorders attributed to work overload, anxiety from fear of toxicity and errors, lack of esteem, and insufficient resources and training in communication skills (Whippen and Canellos 1991; Ramirez et al. 1995). These findings are not unique to oncology. Although research consistently points to communication and relationships with patients as a main source of job satisfaction, physicians suffer from a lack of support services or training in this area. In this context, narrative training through writing and reading may be an ideal method to fight professional "burnout."

As all aspects of medical practice come under greater scrutiny than ever before, it is time to recognize that denying the emotional responses of professionals leads to negative behaviors and emotions. Patient care and professional identity suffer. Statistics demonstrate that the rates for physician depression and suicide are unacceptably high (Center et al. 2003). We must take a critical look at factors that promote this sad and dangerous trend. I would posit that some of the factors leading to depression in medical professionals come from the inability of physicians to safely and effectively share the stressors inherent in caring for the injured, the ill, and the dying. Narrative methods recognize the importance of admitting to and addressing the emotions that naturally occur in the course of caring for patients. Equally relevant is narrative medicine's role in providing a forum for discussion with trusted colleagues, reducing isolation by sharing these emotionally challenging situations.

CONCLUSIONS

There is no question that technical competence is paramount in medical education, but in attempting to increase empathy and develop professionalism, interpersonal competence is equally important. The patient will not benefit from the most highly skilled technical care unless the provider is equipped with the interpersonal skills to join empathically with the patient during care by recognizing the patient's situation. The movements toward patient-centered medicine, biopsychosocial medicine, and end-of-life care have highlighted the importance of health professionals' personal abilities to elicit information about patients' experience of illness, to bear witness to patients' suffering, and to empathically offer themselves as caregivers. These personal abilities constitute true professionalism, defined by qualities of altruism, self-knowledge, and a sense of justice. Clinical literature reveals a consensus around the tenets of professionalism and the personal qualities required for effective patient care, including self-care, personal awareness, reflection, and a capacity to recognize meaning in one's work. Trends toward cynicism and early abandonment of health profession careers can be countered by enabling health professionals to identify, describe, and share meaningful aspects of practice. In the face of the bureaucratization of medical practice and increasingly fragmented subspecialization, health professionals find strength of purpose from authentic relationships with patients as they witness the courage and resilience of patients in their care. It seems straightforward that these goals should be encouraged. What is less clear is how best to help professionals reach those goals both during training and throughout their careers. The use of narrative skills is one simple, time-efficient, and cost-efficient method that can be introduced in medical education and continued throughout a professional career.

Narrative training is not just another medical school course to master with effective study habits or rote memorization. It is not one particular program or method, but rather it is a process and a manner of thinking that is a valuable means of maintaining professionalism and a professional ethic. As a science major I never was a creative writer. Narrative reflection does not require that the physician be a great writer, but rather, a thoughtful one. Having the opportunity to write down ideas that may be plaguing me, and the opportunity to share those ideas, is comforting, supportive, and constructive. Writing itself can provide great solace and relief. Expressing one's thoughts on paper allows the physician to recognize sorrow, and sharing these thoughts helps prevent isolation in a profession where separation is common. Writing about patient experiences has helped me see my patients in a different light. Rather than engaging in talk sessions alone, I have found the process of writing and reading is important because in writing narrative one prepares, refines, and really thinks in depth about the topic (patient, situation, feeling). Forming written words gets to the heart of the matter much sooner than the unformed topic rolling through one's mind and coming to one's lips. Engaging in narrative medicine is not an exercise to improve writing skills. It is a process to acknowledge empathy and our own humanity amidst the necessary demands of distanced professionalism that dominates medical training and practice. The use of narrative methods to share, discuss, and brainstorm on how to improve medical care for ourselves and for our patients is a lifelong initiative to maintain our professional integrity and fight the forces that keep us from providing the type of care we all wish to give and to receive.

REFERENCES

American Board of Internal Medicine (ABIM). 1999. *Project professionalism*. Philadelphia: American Board of Internal Medicine Communications.

Bardes, C. L. 2004. Teaching, digression, and implicit curriculum. *Teaching and Learning in Medicine* 16(2): 212–14.

Benbassat, J., and R. Baumal. 2004. What is empathy, and how can it be promoted during clinical clerkships? *Academic Medicine* 79(9): 832–39.

Brady, D. W., G. Corbie-Smith, and W. T. Branch. 2002. 'What's important to you?' The use of narratives to promote self-reflection and to understand the experiences of medical residents. *Annals of Internal Medicine* 137(3): 220–23.

Branch, W. T., et al. 1993. Becoming a doctor. Critical-incident reports from third-year medical students. *New England Journal of Medicine* 329(15): 1130–32.

Center, C., et al. 2003. Confronting depression and suicide in physicians: A consensus statement. *Journal of the American Medical Association* 289(23): 3161–66.

Charon, R. 2001a. What narrative competence is for. *American Journal of Bioethics* 1(1): 62–63.

———. 2001b. Narrative medicine: form, function, and ethics. *Annals of Internal Medicine* 134(1): 83–87.

———. 2004. Narrative and medicine. *New England Journal of Medicine* 350(9): 862–64.

Coulehan, J. L. 1995. The first patient: Reflections and stories about the anatomy cadaver. *Teaching and Learning in Medicine* 7(1): 61–66.

DasGupta, S., and R. Charon. 2004. Personal illness narratives: Using reflective writing to teach empathy. *Academic Medicine* 79(4): 351–56.

Hatem, D., and E. Ferrara. 2001. Becoming a doctor: Fostering humane caregivers through creative writing. *Patient Education and Counseling* 45: 13–22.

Horowitz, C. R., et al. 2003. What do doctors find meaningful about their work? *Annals of Internal Medicine* 138(9): 772–75.

Kleinman, A. 1988. *The illness narratives: suffering, healing, and the human condition.* New York: Basic Books.

Marshall, P., and O'Keefe, J. P. 1995. Medical students' first-person narratives of a patient's story of AIDS. *Society, Science and Medicine* 40: 67–76.

Maslach, C., W. B. Schaufeli, and M. P. Leiter. 2001. Job burnout. *Annual Review of Psychology* 52: 397–422.

Platt, F. W., et al. 2001. 'Tell me about yourself': The patient-centered interview. *Annals of Internal Medicine* 134(11): 1079–85.

Poirier, S., W. R. Ahrens, and D. J. Brauner. 1998. Songs of innocence and experience: Students' poems about their medical education. *Academic Medicine* 73(5): 473–78.

Ramirez, A. J., et al. 1995. Burnout and psychiatric disorder among cancer clinicians. *British Journal of Cancer* 71(6): 1263–69.

Verghese, A. 2001. The physician as storyteller. *Annals of Internal Medicine* 135(11): 1012–17.

Wear, D., and L. L. Nixon. 2002. Literary inquiry and professional development in medicine: Against abstractions. *Perspectives in Biology and Medicine* 45(1): 104–24.

Whippen, D. A., and G. P. Canellos. 1991. Burnout syndrome in the practice of oncology: Results of a random survey of 1,000 oncologists. *Journal of Clinical Oncology* 9(10): 1916–20.

3

Generational Differences and the Challenges to Achieving a More Reflective Definition for Professionalism

Norma E. Wagoner, Ph.D., and Alison S. Clay, M.D.

At no time in our history have two paired generations with such diversity of values and beliefs been asked to work side by side in such a dynamic medical system. Those in Generations X and Y, who operate with a greater focus on achieving a balanced lifestyle, contrast with those in the oldest working generation (dubbed "veterans") and the baby boomers, who adhere to a more stringent work ethic. The difference in values between these two generational groups has led to a discrepancy in how each perceives those values that constitute professionalism. Academic and societal issues have further complicated the picture as each generation struggles to work through the myriad of changes that have occurred over the past decade. As the medical profession now seeks to define, teach, and assess professionalism, it becomes imperative to understand generational differences, pinpoint the conflicts that have resulted, and, finally, to determine a more reflective definition of professionalism acceptable to all.

As members of the medical community and of different generations, we (authors Wagoner and Clay) have come to appreciate that although Generation X and Y individuals may have different goals and values than their predecessors had, they are no less professional or altruistic. In our ideal vision, the heart of professionalism (truthfulness, adherence to ethical principles, concern for others, and compassion) has not changed throughout the generations. We believe it is crucial for all four generations to desist from the "I'm right, you're wrong" stance and make every effort to accept each other's values and beliefs. To allow the conflict to continue will be to throw out the proverbial baby with the bathwater. In order to graduate the finest possible physicians from medical schools and residency programs, we must put aside our stereotypes and unfounded judgments and strive to find a basis of understanding. The key to success in any conflict lies in negotiation. "Dialogue binds us together as communities . . . it matters a great deal whether we like, respect, trust and understand one another, or stereotype, distance, distort and mistrust one another" (Yankelovich 1999, 4). Throughout this chapter we seek to promote understanding of some generational conflicts by initiating a dialogue between the generations, first by comparing and contrasting the values of each generation of students and physicians, second by exploring the societal and academic challenges they face, and, finally, by discussing each generation's unique response to these challenges as they interact with each other and as they care for patients.

DEFINITION OF THE GENERATIONS

Most sociologists agree that Generation X includes those born between 1960 and 1980. The first to grow up with two working parents, this generation seems to have taken a unanimous vow not to repeat what they regard as their boomer parents' mistake in devoting their lives to their jobs. They saw the economy falter in the mid- to late 1980s, and they watched as their parents were demoted or fired when their employers' companies were "downsized." This experience reshaped their view of loyalty; they dedicate themselves to the job only as long as it meets their needs (Loughlin 2004).

The Y generation (nexters) refers to those born between 1980 and the present. Demographers note that this is one of the largest and most influential groups of individuals to enter the workplace. Generation Y brings more commitment to civic duty, values achievement, and morality, and possesses greater street smarts and a more optimistic outlook than their predecessor generation. Members of Generation Y are the most techno-savvy to come along, which gives them what they feel is an authoritative edge. Although minor differences occur between these generations, they retain many similarities in values, with their quest for work-life balance being central among them.

The loyalties of these younger generations revolve to a great extent around themselves and their friends and families rather than their jobs. According to Moody (2004), this group works to live rather than lives to work. She cites eight general characteristics of this group: (1) more likely to be female; (2) hold lifestyle as a core concern; (3) seek immediate stability; (4) do not seek hierarchical dominance; (5) technically savvy; (6) have skills-based mind-set; (7) loyal to principles, not organizations; and (8) seek conflict resolution. Members of Generations X and Y view the practice of medicine as a profession, not a lifestyle; they intend to have time for family and social interaction outside their professions. They prefer group practice or hospital employment with built-in structure (defined practice hours, limited call, reasonable patient loads), assistance in relief from educational debt, and a secure, guaranteed salary.

The so-called "veteran" generation loosely encompasses those born between 1922 and 1943, while the baby boomer generation consists of those born between 1944 and 1960. As a broad generalization, it can be said that individuals in these generations share similar values in their adherence to the Christian work ethic, based on delayed gratification and unremitting toil. Most physicians from this generation place their patients' needs above their own and those of their families and friends. They have always put their profession first, even if it has meant long hours and personal sacrifice. These physicians have and continue to define themselves first and foremost as doctors.

CONFLICT OF VALUES

For many years, veterans and baby boomers served as faculty members and administrators for medical students and residents who belonged to the same generations. With this alignment of values and beliefs, the concept of professionalism rarely came into question. Unfortunately, this is no longer the situation.

In recent years, medical schools have experienced a large influx of students with diverse ethnic and cultural backgrounds, and an increasing number of women. The social and cultural mores of these groups often deviate significantly from the traditional standards of professionalism used by the older generation in their evaluation and teaching. Older physicians have difficulty dealing with the younger generations' priorities: their commitment to cultural values, to family, and to a life outside of practice. With the disparity in generational values, attitudes, and behaviors, faculty members frequently face significant challenges and frustrations in their job of educating and mentoring. They watch in astonishment as members of the younger generation struggle throughout their education and training to balance careers and family, and they may perceive this balancing of priorities as indicative of a lack of accountability, responsibility, and professionalism. A survey of physicians fifty to sixty-five years old found older physicians to be disillusioned with the young generation; when asked whether the respondents considered their young counterparts as dedicated and hardworking as they were, 100 percent of respondents said "no" (Rogers-Stokes 2004, 2).

Generation X and Y medical students and physician trainees also struggle with generational differences. Today's students and residents exhibit different behavioral norms in many respects: how they learn, solve problems, communicate, interact with authority figures, develop goals, and, in general, conduct their daily activities (Lahiri 2001). They expect to find a life-work balance while simultaneously achieving professional success. They do not hesitate to look for alternatives if they feel their personal time or freedom is being significantly hindered. The younger generations have grown up with and mastered rapidly changing technology. They recognize their technical proficiency as superior to those of the older generation, giving them an edge in the increasingly computerized world of practice. They tend to judge as antiquated the hierarchical model of moving up within an organization and insist that those in the veteran/boomer generation acknowledge their technical proficiency by treating them more as colleagues. Imbedded in this technology-driven mind-set is an expectation of rapid change and immediate payback. Kennedy captures this characteristic: "Managing different generations requires new skills, insightful leadership—Gen X is here!" Generation X and Y physicians do not subscribe to the idea of "paying their dues, having their ideas ignored or told to wait until they've learned more about the organizational culture. If the job lacks content or the break-in period is too long before any real challenges emerge, they are gone and quick to say why" (Kennedy 2003, 5).

Operating on their own set of values, Generation X and Y trainees perceive their outlook and actions as professional and don't understand the older generations' frustration.

Conflicting attitudes toward priorities, whether based on gender, race, or cultural or generational differences, have resulted in an "us against them" split between generations, commensurate with resentments that stifle productivity and destroy team spirit, a critical aspect of medicine.

In an effort to initiate a dialogue that could lead to a modicum of resolution, we will explore how each generation reacts to the ever-increasing number of challenges posed by changes in the field of medicine, the academic environment, and the desire for controllable lifestyle careers.

CHALLENGE I: THE CHANGING FACE OF MEDICINE

Thirty years ago, the typical family doctor (a majority were men at that time) ordinarily spent his entire career in one town. He had extensive knowledge of each patient and that patient's family. He most likely shared the same values as the rest of the town's residents and was entrusted with making decisions for patients and their families. Doctors were on call twenty-four hours a day, seven days a week; physicians placed the needs of their patients first, often at the expense of their own families. In return, the doctor received tremendous satisfaction in helping his patients, and he and his family were respected members of the community.

Tremendous change has occurred in the practice of medicine in the past few decades, both in terms of scientific advances and in the management, reimbursement, and societal expectations of medicine. As recently as 1960, physicians could offer sick patients far fewer medical interventions than are available today. A patient with a myocardial infarction might be admitted for two weeks for bed rest, while today that same patient might receive powerful medications, undergo invasive techniques, and even be supported indefinitely by mechanical means while waiting for a heart transplant.

The increasingly invasive nature and technical advances of medicine have given rise to unique problems. Physicians must train longer and harder to master clinical skills through continued fellowship training. Not only have subspecialties emerged, so have regional geographic areas of expertise. Physician trainees must fully comprehend the physical, metabolic, and chemical alterations induced by today's medicine in order to prevent patients from suffering ill effects or dying. They also must know to whom they can refer patients and when to do it.

The myriad of changes over the past several decades has led to a dramatic shift in the public's expectation of health care delivery. Patients have come to believe that there is a treatment for every medical problem, that life support is a valid option, and that medication exists for every ailment. And they want their care now. Patients have easy access to medical knowledge; with the click of a mouse they can research their health problems, determine possible diagnoses and treatments, and demand the treatment they feel is necessary. Public attention to the dangers of medicine, such as those revealed in the Institute of Medicine's reports "To Err is Human" and "Crossing the Quality Chasm," have added additional skepticism to the doctor-patient relationship (IOM 1998; IOM 2001). Understandably, today's physicians cannot always meet their patients' expectations. If a physician does not offer the patient the course of treatment she wants in the time frame she wants it, the patient will likely seek a second or third opinion or help from a different specialist. As a result, most patients have transient relationships with more than one physician, and may see physicians outside their geographic locale, thus further eroding the doctor-patient relationship.

Simultaneously, the cost of health care has increased at rates that seem exponential to medical advances. In the past four decades, health care has seen the emergence of managed care, introduced to defray some of the costs of medicine. Physicians have been asked to attend both to the patient and the insurance company. To complete paperwork and meet patient load demands, physicians have been forced to decrease patient contact time. The loss of contact time has resulted in additional consumer/patient dissatisfaction. In this era in which patients demand more of physicians in terms of care, treatments, and accessibility, they have had to settle for less, and their trust in and respect for doctors and the medical profession as a whole has greatly diminished.

Fischman describes the current strain on the doctor-patient relationship thus: "It is no longer a happy marriage, this relationship between doctors and patients. A bond once tight with intimacy is under incredible strain. Doctors have changed. Patients have changed. The caring is gone. Well, not gone but buried under the crush of everyday life. Buried under insurance headaches as patients now come burdened with reams of paperwork for doctors to fill out for reimbursement, paperwork that eats away at the time they might spend on other patients" (Fischman 2005, 46).

The collision of public expectations with a struggling health care system has resulted in skyrocketing malpractice rates, particularly since 1999. By 2004, the medical liability insurance industry was losing $1.53 for every $1.00 collected (PIAA 2004). Insurance premiums rose as a result of these losses, making it impossible in some states for physicians to obtain liability insurance in high-risk fields such as neurosurgery, obstetrics, emergency medicine, and radiology (Mello 2003). Studdert et al. discuss five plausible explanations for the increasing frequency and size of liability payouts: "greater public awareness of medical errors; lower levels of confidence and trust in the health care system among patients as a result of negative experiences with managed care; advances in medical innovation particularly diagnostic technology and increases in the intensity of medical services; rising public expectations about medical care and finally, a greater reluctance among plaintiffs' attorneys to accept offers that in the past would have closed cases" (Studdert et al. 2004, 285).

Public dissatisfaction and lack of trust have taken a toll on physicians' attitudes. A 2001 California survey found that 75 percent of physician respondents indicated less satisfaction with practicing medicine over the previous five years (Hobson 2005). In a survey of physicians fifty to sixty-five years old, the majority of respondents related "general dissatisfaction with today's medical practice environment" (Rogers-Stokes 2004, 2). Trainees are also less satisfied. A 2003 survey of residents asked whether they would study medicine or select another field if they had their education to begin again; 25 percent said they would select another field, compared to less than 5 percent when surveyed two years before (Merritt, Hawkins, and Associates 2003).

What was once considered central in the reward system for physicians in practicing medicine—satisfying relationships with patients, autonomy, high status, and comparatively high pay—has been replaced in greater measure with volumes of paperwork, declining reimbursements, loss of autonomy, and fear of malpractice suits. Unquestionably the intensity and style of medicine have changed, and the changes have had far-reaching effects—altering the academic and learning environments, affecting career choices, increasing attrition rates, and raising questions about what has happened to the professionalism that existed in earlier days.

CHALLENGE II: THE CHANGING ACADEMIC ENVIRONMENT IN RESIDENCY PROGRAMS

The academic environment has changed substantially in residency programs. A veteran's or a boomer's training to become a physician consisted primarily of an apprenticeship carried out with a few master clinicians. Because the trainee lived in the hospital, house staff and faculty members knew each other well and fewer external distractions arose relevant to raising a family or managing a household. Although they were in a hierarchical system, the trainee and physician had personal investments in each other: the attending physician invested time in the trainee, who was expected to "pay back" either by doing "scut" during residency or by mentoring others in the style of his mentor after residency. Years after they have completed their training, veteran and boomer trainees frequently speak fondly of their mentors. This training model has been replaced with one that is far less personal and more transient; residents do not live in the hospital, take call less frequently, and work with a larger number of faculty members. These changes have evolved as a result of both more intense medicine and new regulations for residency training.

In response to public attention on medical errors and patient safety, in 2003 the Accreditation Council for Graduate Medical Education (ACGME) instituted several new work rules for residents. The rules limit residents' hours to fewer than eighty per week averaged over a four-week period, and restricted call periods to no more than every third night. In addition, residents may not work continuously for more than twenty-four hours, plus six hours for transitions in patient care.

These regulations, while critical in the overall care of patients, have had significant repercussions in residency programs. Residents feel torn between following the rules and taking care of their patients. Although residents realize that the rules were established for patient safety and that they should abide by them, doing so appears to compete with the care they feel dedicated to provide. David Leach, M.D., executive director of the ACGME, describes the dilemma that residents face: "Residents have depended on vigilance . . . knowing that the system can't be trusted. Now we've reduced the availability of the residents, and they are worried. They want to stay [at the hospital] because they can't trust the system." Thus, rather than abiding by regulations designed to protect them, residents find ways to go around them, often violating the spirit of the eighty-hour work week rules by fudging the monthly logs about the number of hours they work (Croasdale 2004a, 2).

If residents manage to limit their work hours to eighty hours per week, they face consternation from their supervisors. Those attending physicians who lack familiarity with or do not accept the new training rules may view residents as lazy or uncommitted to their patients and therefore lacking critical professional ethics. At a recent conference, author Wagoner heard a physician near her own age comment that the "shift work mentality" of trainees causes him great concern. He remarked on how much more difficult it is now to find the kind of commitment to patients that physicians in his day considered paramount to their role as professionals. "Older attending physicians worked unending hours as residents, and the new work rules don't fit in with their idea of professionalism." Residents are keenly aware of this attitude. He quoted a resident as saying, "It's not cool to leave, to just sign out, you are seen as irresponsible if you leave" (Croasdale 2004b, 3).

When comparing themselves to the current house staff, faculty physicians may not take into consideration how dramatically the training system has changed. In their frustration with the new regulations, they often misdirect their anger and bitterness toward the trainees, failing to remember that the residents did not instigate the work hour limitation rules and, as previously mentioned, often try to avoid them. In addition, these faculty members may not be aware that although current residents generally have less frequent call responsibilities, call periods differ significantly from those the attending physicians experienced in their training. In a study evaluating how residents spend call time, Thomas (2005) noted that while residents spent every other night on call in 1960, they spent 7.5 hours in their call rooms each night. In contrast, in 1990, residents spent 4.5 hours per night in their call room, and in 2003 only 1.7 hours. In the same study, Thomas also noted that residents' time spent on patient care varied dramatically, with residents in 2003 devoting almost 30 percent of their time tracking down, following, and documenting patient data on the computer. Residents now often obtain complicated patient histories from an electronic record rather than from talking to the patients in person. This time spent away from patients may contribute to the less personal relationship attending physicians have witnessed between residents and patients (Thomas 2005).

Many of the regulations and changes have altered the doctor-patient relationship. As residents spend more time at the computers and less time with patients, they do not have the opportunity to develop personal relationships with patients. When residents leave at the end of the imposed thirty-hour period, they must transition care to other residents, physician extenders, or their attending physician. Not only does this handing off add additional strain on the attending faculty physician, who must spend time covering the residents, it limits both the resident-attending contact time and the resident-patient contact time. It is not surprising that some residents come to feel diminished accountability for or commitment to patient care.

At the same time the ACGME instituted work hours, it introduced six general domains of behavior or competencies residents must demonstrate prior to graduation. With this formalization of the education process, residents may need to leave patient care to participate in simulations, standardized patient encounters, and learning workshops. As residents spend less, more fragmented time in patient care, not only are their relationships with the patients at risk, but so too are their relationships with their mentors. Residents still want and need enthusiastic role models. They count on their mentors to teach them medical and surgical techniques, to assist in their personal development, and to help negotiate their work-life balance.

In the current training environment, these expectations prove unrealistic; faculty members simply lack the time to devote to intensive mentoring. They have to balance increased teaching and clinical supervision responsibilities with escalating administrative requirements. Attending physicians also face the demands of increased public scrutiny on individual and hospital outcomes for procedures. Although faculty members spend less time with each resident and thus fail to gain familiarity with his or her strengths and weaknesses, they are still expected to provide residents with learning opportunities and procedural experiences. These multiple administrative and resident demands may constrain an attending physician's ability to maintain excellent clinical outcome data. Coupled with their frustration over trying to meet multiple obligations, faculty members may harbor the feeling that residents are working less, are less accountable, less responsible, and less willing to "pay back" the attending physician.

Not only has the relationship between residents and attending physicians been eroded, relationships between the doctors and their patients have generally become more transient and less satisfying for all. The loss of close interaction produces considerable tension as each generation tries to meet the needs and expectations of the other and of society as well, and ultimately feel they fall short in both areas. The most profound outcome of the institution of ACGME regulations is the realization that there is simply too much work for too few doctors.

CHALLENGE III: CAREER CHOICES

Whether the result of changes in the field of medicine, medical school and training experiences, and/or gender and cultural diversity, students today are making drastically different career choices than their supervisors, and they are making them for different reasons. These career choices and the reasons behind them serve to augment intergenerational conflict.

In keeping with their desire to devote themselves to lives of service, veteran and boomer physicians tended to choose specialties based on intellectual and personal strengths that would enable them to make a difference in the health and welfare of the patients they hoped to serve. Certainly many Generation X and Y medical students also base their career choices in part on these virtues, but they also place greater emphasis on selecting specialties that enable them to both maintain a balanced lifestyle and do well financially. In 1999, Petrie and colleagues surveyed 520 medical students from the University of Auckland Medical School (258 men and 262 women) about the important driving forces in their lives. The top four responses to a question asking for three top wishes were: (1) happiness with my career and personal life (34 percent), (2) money (32 percent), (3) altruism (helping others in need) (31 percent), and (4) achievement (to become a top specialist) (27 percent) (Petrie 1999). This study shows that priorities between generations have virtually reversed.

Several other studies also show that Generation X and Y students consider altruism less important in their career selection than did their veteran and boomer predecessors. In 1990, Schwartz et al. asked 346 fourth-year students from nine medical schools about influences in their career choices. Analysis of responses to their questionnaire revealed three groups of influences: perceived lifestyle (remuneration, personal time, and prestige), cerebral activities and practice orientation, and altruistic values and attitudes. The authors then classified the medical students' actual career choices into three groups: noncontrollable lifestyle—NCL (internal medicine, family practice, pediatrics, and obstetrics and gynecology); controllable lifestyle—CL (anesthesiology, dermatology, emergency medicine, neurology, ophthalmology, otolaryngology, pathology, psychiatry, and radiology); and surgery (also an NCL for which the authors sought specific information because of their special interest). They found that students choosing careers in the controllable lifestyle group were the least influenced by altruistic values and attitudes, while students choosing the NCL specialties scored highest in altruism (Schwartz 1990).

Another study by Barclay corroborates the Schwartz finding: "They [Generation X and Y] are thinking, if I can be a radiologist or emergency medicine doctor and train for half the time commitment, be finished with training at a younger age, potentially make two times as much in salary, and have a lot more free time, well I don't care about that exhilaration in the operating room; I'd rather have the extra time and extra money to enjoy things outside of work" (Barclay 2004, 2). Despite their ordering of priorities, we do not believe that the younger generations lack the values of altruism; they simply express these values differently. For example, when trainees spend time with their patients, they are fully vested in their patients' interests and outcomes, and when they are with their families, they give them full measure of their attention.

The influx of women has contributed significantly to the selection of controllable lifestyle careers. Women who entered medicine in the 1990s and after tended to choose specialties that allow them a greater degree of flexibility. Research has shown that women hold more than 50 percent of the positions in residency programs in family practice, psychiatry, dermatology, pediatrics, and obstetrics and gynecology, specialties that by and large have granted them greater opportunity to achieve the balanced lifestyle they desire (Moody 2004). Women also may choose careers with a more controllable lifestyle in order to have and raise a family. "The link between women's education and delayed childbirth has been well established. For women with 16+ years of education, median age at first birth rose by 3.8 years to 29.5 between 1969 and 1994, with 45.5% of first births among those women occurring at age 30 or older, quadrupling the rate found in 1969" (Barnett et al. 2003).

External factors also contribute to career choices. Merritt, Hawkins, et al., in their 2003 survey of final-year residents, noted that more than 60 percent of resident respondents expressed significant concern regarding rising malpractice insurance rates and the effects of managed health care. The authors concluded, "It is easy to infer, therefore, that residents will be seeking practice opportunities that can alleviate their concerns, including opportunities both low in malpractice and in low managed care areas" (Merritt, Hawkins and Associates 2003, 6).

Many of the specialties with a controllable lifestyle carry less liability risk because the patients' expectations may be met more easily. In radiology, dermatology, or anesthesiology, for example, specific boundaries limit the proffered services, the accessibility of the physician, and the length of the doctor-patient relationship. For instance, a patient expects her anesthesiologist to put her to sleep and thus does not anticipate a long-term relationship with that physician or to have accessibility to that physician beyond the perioperative period. Since the physician can meet the expectations of the patient, both are satisfied with the encounter. An additional benefit is that patient satisfaction has been shown to reduce malpractice rates (Forster et al. 2002; Levinson et al. 1997).

Although it may not be evident to the veteran or boomer generations, Generation X and Y individuals look forward to many of the same rewards the veterans and boomers sought years ago—not only financial reward, but respect from patients and a feeling of having done a good job. For today's trainees, these rewards may be more attainable in different specialties than those chosen by the veterans and boomers.

CHALLENGE IV: COMPETITION AND ATTRITION

Competition in medical school and residency programs contributes to the differing values, expectations, and behaviors of Generation X and Y students and residents. Not only do students compete to get into the very best medical schools, they face serious competition later in obtaining residency positions that guarantee their preferred lifestyle. This fierce competition may restrict students' ability to attain life-enriching experiences, thus reducing or eliminating risk-taking endeavors that have the potential to negatively impact their transcripts. This in turn limits students' moral development and awareness of personal values and robs them of the opportunity to explore interests both inside and outside of medicine. All told, students may not have nurtured altruistic values nor come to an understanding of which specialty best suits their goals. A lesser yet significant outcome is that with a lack of life experiences and risk-taking endeavors, students often fail to develop coping skills essential for the clinical years and residency.

The delay in medical students' and residents' personal, emotional, and moral development poses significant challenges for matching a student to the appropriate residency, as well as for filling residencies with appropriately qualified residents. With little time to fully explore career options, students may choose a field that has more demands or is less fulfilling than they expected, and/or does not support important priorities and values to which they subscribe. As more and more students and residents choose specialties with controllable lifestyles, the other, often larger, specialties lose the most qualified residents. As the number and quality of students pursuing careers in internal medicine and surgery drop, it seems less likely that society's expectations of medicine can be met, either because there won't be enough physicians in those fields or because those who are there may be less committed due to their lack of success in entering the fields they desired (Richtel 2004).

Strong competition can result in residents "defaulting" into specialties that do not offer the lifestyles they wanted. The resulting mismatch between physician desires and patient/residency needs can lead to attrition. In a 2002 survey, 25 to 30 percent of program director respondents in surgery, family medicine, and internal medicine agreed that attrition was a national problem. Reasons directors cited for attrition included: (1) being unprepared for the work demands of graduate medical education; (2) never really committed to the specialty; and (3) wanted to stay at home and raise a family or be with their family. In all, 44 percent of program directors attributed the loss of residents to other specialties over a period of three years to (ranked highest to lowest) (1) insufficient understanding of the specialty chosen, (2) personality not suited for the specialty, (3) could not reconcile specialty demands with personal life, and (4) demands of the specialty would interfere with desires for lifestyle (Wagoner and Suriano 2002).

Attending physicians who have chosen a particular specialty for altruistic or academic reasons experience frustration working with dissatisfied residents who have no desire to be in that specialty. Residency program directors, trying to accommodate the residents' search for their final career path, spend a great deal of time and energy searching for alternate training for unhappy residents and for replacements for departing residents. Attending faculty members and directors may feel used by residents who lack commitment to their training or who fail to acknowledge the time, effort, and expense that has been spent on them. While the resident has demanded assistance and commitment from the program, attending physicians and directors often feel that residents have not proffered the same level of commitment. These challenges likely will continue as graduating medical students and residents enter the workforce and continue to seek a balanced lifestyle and a fulfilling career.

CHALLENGE V: THE LEARNING ENVIRONMENT

Medical education starts, or should start, with the selection of those applicants committed to becoming competent and compassionate physicians. The medical school then assumes the responsibility of reinforcing students' values of professionalism along with teaching them technical proficiency—a duality that has been recognized since the turn of the twentieth century. Thus, it becomes incumbent upon medical schools to combat the disturbing effects of competition, including delayed moral development and a lack of commitment or responsibility. It goes without saying that medical schools also should nurture altruism, service, and empathy, values central to the goal of becoming a professional. In his autobiography, Abraham Flexner wrote, "Medical education is not just a program of building knowledge and skills in its recipients . . . it is also about experience that creates attitudes and expectations" (Flexner 1960). Unfortunately, research studies show that the learning environment not only fails to develop these professional attributes, it also contributes to a decline in students' moral values. Jordan Cohen, M.D., outgoing president of the Association of American Medical Colleges, states, "Unless we can convert our learning environments from crucibles of cynicism into cradles of professionalism, no amount of effort in the admissions arena is going to suffice" (Cohen 2002).

Several studies indicate that moral development, altruism, and empathy suffer during medical school and residency training. Patenaude et al. assessed progress in moral development in medical students by examining the ethical development of students during their medical education years. The authors "did not observe the increase in the development of moral reasoning that was expected . . . [but instead] found a significant decrease in weighted average scores after three years of medical education" (Patenaude et al. 2003).

What contributes to the decline in values? The consensus of research suggests that students and residents acquire their values from the mentors they observe during medical school and residency. Students observe the mind-sets, moral stances, and hour-to-hour decisions made by authority figures. From these encounters, students learn how to best use their time, how and what to think and feel, and how to solve problems. This implicit curriculum, dubbed the "hidden curriculum," has been found to play a significant role in the formation of trainees. Stern (1998) states that trainees acquire the humanistic values inherent in the hidden curriculum during call, late at night. In a study of longitudinal changes in mood and empathy over the course of the internal medicine residency, Bellini et al. concluded that challenges for medical educators largely consist of "protecting the development of empathy during times of immense change" (Bellini and Shea 2005, 167).

CHALLENGE VI: DEFINING, TEACHING, AND ASSESSING PROFESSIONALISM

No one can doubt the importance of teaching and evaluating professionalism in medicine. However, the changes in the practice of medicine and in the training of physicians raise several questions about professionalism. Is it possible to teach a common set of attitudes and values to students and residents of diverse cultures and ethnic backgrounds? Assuming that professionalism can be taught, who would appropriately teach the attitudes and values encompassed within the models adopted by the medical schools and residencies?

Defining, teaching, and assessing professionalism to accommodate public expectations in fairness to both sets of generations will not be an easy task. Nevertheless, we believe it can be accomplished through a combination of innovation, pragmatism, and willingness to dispense with the way things have always been done. In order to be successful in the twenty-first century, medical schools and residency programs must diligently strive to create a learning environment that includes and supports the wide spectrum of cultural differences, norms, and styles. A careful assessment should be undertaken as to what is being taught in the explicit curriculum as well as in the hidden and null curriculum at both medical school and residency levels. Faculty physicians must be called upon to nurture medical students and residents by modeling empathy and altruism and by assisting them to achieve their ideal vision. We cannot overemphasize the role of mentoring for both students and residents. One solution resides in promoting less transient, longer lasting relationships between faculty members and residents. In knowing a resident well, including his or her deficiencies, faculty members come to understand better the resident's values and are less likely to interpret his or her behavior as unprofessional. Medical schools and residency programs can do a great deal to promote faculty-student and faculty-resident relationships, both by reducing the multiple demands on faculty members' time and thoroughly familiarizing them with the many new training and medical education rules. In residency programs, one possible solution could be greater use of clinician-educators who know the residents well and have complete knowledge of training regulations.

First and foremost, however, medical schools and residency programs must come to a clear understanding and acceptance of disparate generational values. Rather than simply perceiving the values of Generations X and Y as "deficient," faculty members and directors should consider defining the stereotypes and biases of each generation, then factoring these definitions into the creation of a more reflective definition by which to evaluate professional attitudes and behaviors.

Conversely, it becomes incumbent upon students and residents to consider and make allowances for differing values held by faculty members and directors. Formal and informal focused discussions with faculty members and directors could help elucidate differences. Such discussions will require careful, thoughtful communication geared toward reducing resentment and bringing accord into the personal and working relationship between the generational groups.

CONCLUSION

We hope this chapter has succeeded in raising awareness of generational differences and the challenges that have compounded these differences. The assumption that your values as the student/resident are the same as my values as the administrator/professor/program director no longer holds true, and a new model must be created to replace it. We believe that despite their determination to protect a portion of their waking hours for their families, friends, and outside activities, young physicians will find a way to give their patients the best possible care. We do not subscribe to the notion that self-interest serves as the enemy of altruism. As students and residents, young physicians overcome tremendous competition. As residents, they bypass regulations to assure their patients' safety. Does it not follow then that they will continue to do whatever it takes to ensure their patients' well-being? We believe they will. We believe it is time for the differing generations to engage in what can be described as the "process of dialogue that binds us together as communities" (Yankelovich 1999). Working together on a more reflective definition of professionalism not only will better serve patients, but it will bring the community of medicine more in accord with its moral obligation to those it seeks to serve.

Once we take time to appreciate each other's values, we will come to realize that those in every generation maintain an unwavering commitment to the patient that simply manifests differently. It is in fact the patient who bridges the generations and who will ultimately compel a resolution of generational conflicts. If we renew our focus on the patient and take advantage of each generation's unique skills, we can continue to expand the frontiers of science as well as the art of medicine. For all our differences, this commitment to the patient is sacrosanct, binding physicians from the time of Hippocrates to today and into the future.

REFERENCES

Accreditation Council for Graduate Medical Education (ACGME). 1999. The ACGME Outcome Project: General Competencies [cited 18 November 2005]. Available from www.acgme.org/outcome/comp/compFull.asp.

Barclay, L. 2004. Surgery less popular as a career choice, a newsmaker interview with Susan Brundage, M.D. *Medscape, Medical News* [cited 29 June 2004]. Available: www.medscape.com/viewarticle/481415.

Barnett R. C., K. C. Gareis, J. B. James, and J. Steele. 2003. Planning Ahead: College seniors' concerns about career-marriage conflict. *Journal of Vocational Behavior* 62: 305–19.

Bellini, L., and J. Shea. 2005. Mood change in empathy decline persists during three years of internal medicine training. *Academic Medicine* 80(2): 164–67.

Cohen, J. 2002. Our compact with tomorrow's doctors. *Academic Medicine* 77(6): 475–79.

Croasdale, M. 2004a. Beat the clock: the new challenges to residents. *AMANews*. March 8, 2004 [cited 12 July 2004]. Available: www.ama-assn.org/amednews/2004/03/08prsa0308.htm.

———. 2004b. Resident work-hour limits still a struggle one year into restrictions. *AMANews*. July 19, 2004 [cited 22 July 2004]. Available: www.ama-assn.org/amednews/2004/07/19prl10719.htm.

Fischman, J. 2005. Who will take care of you? *US News and World Report*. January 31–February 7: 46.

Flexner, A. 1960. *Abraham Flexner: An Autobiography*. New York: Simon and Schuster.

Forster, H., et al. 2002. Reducing legal risk by practicing patient-centered medicine. *Archives of Internal Medicine* 162(11): 1217–19.

Hobson, K. 2005. Doctors vanish from view. *US News and World Report*. January 31–February 7: 48.

Institute of Medicine (IOM). 1998. Linda T. Kohn et al. To Err Is Human: Building a Safer Health System. Washington, D.C.: Institute of Medicine.

———. 2001. Crossing the Quality Chasm: A New Health System for the 21st Century. Washington, D.C.: Institute of Medicine.

Kennedy, M. 2003. Managing different generations requires new skills, insightful leadership—Gen X is here! *Physician Executive*, Nov–Dec 2003.

Lahiri, I. 2001. *Understanding and addressing intergenerational conflict*. Workforce Development Group. The GilDeane Group, published May 15, 2001 [cited 5 January 2005]. Available: www.workforcedevelopmentgroup.com/news_ninteen.html.

Levinson, W., et al. 1997. Physician-patient communication. Relationship with malpractice claims among primary care physicians and surgeons. *Journal of the American Medical Association* 277(7): 553–59.

Loughlin, C. 2004. Changes in the workplace: Today's young workers become tomorrow's workforce. *Management and Economics Review* 1(2) [cited 19 July 2004]. Available: www.utsc.utoronto.ca/~mgmt/journalvol1no2/loughlin.html.

Mello, M. M., et al. 2003. The new medical malpractice crisis. *New England Journal of Medicine* 348(23): 2281–84.

Merritt, Hawkins & Associates. 2003. *Summary Report: 2003 Survey of Final-year medical residents* [cited 5 January 2005]. Available: www.merritthawkins.com.

Moody, J. 2004. Recruiting generation x physicians. *The New England Journal of Medicine*. Career Center for Employers [cited 5 January 2005]. Available: www.nejmjobs.org/rpt/rpt_article_21.asp.

Patenaude, J., T. Niyonsenga, and D. Fafard. 2003. Changes in students' moral development during medical school: a cohort study. *Canadian Medical Association Journal* 168(7): 840–44.

Petrie, J., et al. 1999. Photographic memory, money, and liposuction: Survey of medical students wish lists. *British Medical Journal* 319: 1593–95.

Physicians Insurers Association of America (PIAA). 2004. "Statement of the PIAA as presented before the joint hearing of the United States Senate Judiciary Committee." February 11, 2004. Available: thepiaa.org/pdf_files/February_11_Testimony/pdf.

Richtel, M. 2004. Young doctors and wish lists: No weekend calls, no beepers. *New York Times.* January 2004 [cited 7 January 2004]. Available: query.nytimes.com/gst/fullpage.html?sec=health&res=9F0DE3DC1031F934A35752C 0A9629C8B63.

Rogers-Stokes, L. 2004. My Generation: Bridging gaps in approach to work, life. *Physicians Practice* [cited 5 January 2005]. Available: www.physicianspractice .com/index.cfm?fuseaction=articles.details&articleID=531.

Schwartz, R., et al. 1990. The controllable lifestyle factor and students' attitudes about specialty selection. *Academic Medicine* 65(9): 207–10.

Stern, D. 1998. Practicing what we preach? An analysis of the curriculum values in medical education. *American Journal of Medicine* 104(6): 605–6.

Studdert, D. M., et al. 2004. Medical Malpractice. *New England Journal of Medicine* 350(3): 283–92.

Thomas, K. 2005. Resident time analysis study: The effect of ACGME duty hour regulations on resident work hour activity. Synderman Award Presentation. ICGME meeting, Duke University, May 11, 2005.

Tobin, M. 2004. Mentoring: Seven roles and some specifics. *American Journal of Respiratory and Critical Care Medicine* 170: 114–17.

Wagoner, N., and J. Suriano. 2002. Patterns and trends: Program directors' perception of residents leaving medicine, changing programs or changing specialties. Unpublished data.

Yankelovich, D. 1999. Having it all. *INC.* September [cited 5 January 2005]. Available: www.inc.com/magazine/19990901/12114.html.

LEARNING PROFESSIONALISM

As professionals (both those formally in training and those engaged in subsequent lifelong development) reflect on the process of becoming professionals, they tend to have particular formative experiences. Often these experiences cause them to reflect on negative role modeling, intense patient encounters, or their personal experiences as patients. Professionals in development, then, can learn as much from experience as from didactic opportunities. Reflection on these experiences is a fundamental aspect of maximizing the internalization of professional ideals observed (or lacking) in the practice environment. The following reflections explore trainees' experiences with patients and colleagues that have influenced their professional development.

4

The Future of Medicine: A Reflection on Medical Professionalism from Future Medical School Students

Justin M. List and Christian J. Krautkramer

Upon a routine visit to his doctor, a young man noticed a new sign: "Copayments are due at the time of check-in. Thank you for your co-operation." Something about this message disturbed him—why was it at this doctor's office that a patient's first interaction was financial? In a way, it was like having the doctor come out and say, "Good morning, open your wallet and I'll be right with you." What troubled him was not the concept of a copayment itself but a perception that money was the doctor's primary interest, as important as his patient's well-being.

Does such a perception put the patient-physician relationship on shaky ground? For patients, would seeing a sign like this encourage them to view the practice of medicine primarily as a business encounter? How much worse could the already ill patient feel if he or she did not have the money that day, regardless if he or she would have it later? Is the potential for making the patient feel momentarily more uncomfortable ethically justified in this type of situation? It is unlikely that a patient would be denied care on the basis of not paying the copayment before the visit, and certainly physicians have prudential and reasonable financial concerns, but it seems unreasonable for the physician to put the patient in this position. Collecting copayments *after* a visit seems a preferable choice on both symbolic and psychological grounds.

If only it were that simple. The man later learned that an insurance company required the posting of this sign. Curious about the insurance company's motivation, he began a conversation with two office assistants. One of them was troubled by the sign because of the possibility for awkward interactions with patients. The other articulated that the sign was justified because of financial concerns; the physician's office would have trouble collecting payment from the insurance company if copays were not received or simply arrived late.

The patient in the above story is one of the coauthors, Justin. Currently a medical student and former medical ethics fellow, Justin decided that a sign requesting money before receiving medical services presented a significant ethical concern to the practice of medicine. Had the business of medicine encroached upon the doctor-patient relationship in a problematic way here? A few years ago, he would have been much less sensitive. After all, on the day of the visit he had good insurance and a low copayment, and the appointment was routine. Even though this was a seemingly small issue in the scope of larger health care issues, Justin's recent education in professionalism gave him pause on this particular practice. We coauthors decided to write our reflections on this issue. We share both the desire to become physicians and the interest in ethics, having met in fellowship training.

Think back to your childhood. Did you ever say, "I want to be a [insert occupation] when I grow up?" How did you arrive at that conclusion? For some of us, that dream was to become a doctor. Where did the inspiration for that dream arise? A simple answer might be our society's high valuation of "professional" occupations such as medicine, occupations valued largely for their altruism and what they "give back" to society. Supreme Court Justice Louis Brandeis once suggested that professional occupations are "pursued largely for others, and not merely for one's own self; and in which the financial return is not the accepted measure of success." For centuries in Western society, those occupations have included religious ministry, law, and medicine. There are many other professions that offer the opportunity to make more money or offer more power and influence. But for those entering the medical profession, the choice often hinges on an apparent and immediate opportunity for daily altruistic action.

Individuals usually prize health above all other things. We frequently hear the adage, "You don't have anything unless you have your health." It is difficult for anyone who is not healthy to lead a flourishing life. Those in the medical profession experience the satisfaction of seeing clear outcomes to their work that help others live their lives more fully, while at the same time receiving a comfortable income. What becomes troubling is when members of the medical profession themselves have poor experiences that create such an unfavorable view of the profession that gifted and talented individuals are discouraged from entering it. The mixing of the "practice of medicine" with the "business of medicine" has often reflected poorly on the medical profession and in many ways has discouraged some from entering it.

Recently, Christian had a conversation with a physician highly respected for his social activism and bedside manner. In the course of the conversation, Christian told this physician that when he revealed his interest in becoming a physician to other physicians, almost everyone responded, "Don't go into medicine. It's awful now." These doctors proceeded to list reasons for the profession's decline: the rise of managed care, increased and unnecessary government oversight, and extravagant costs associated with malpractice protection. The physician responded in kind, "Well, I think that those people are just stupid. It's doctors like those who shouldn't be practicing medicine in the first place." He then proceeded to play devil's advocate: "Okay, fine. Don't go into medicine. There's too much paperwork. Insurance premiums are too high. Doctors don't get to talk to patients anymore and medical practice is commodified to a point where an office visit is like going to the bank. What do you say?" It can be a difficult argument to fight.

We will be entering medical school after employment in the Ethics Group of the American Medical Association (AMA). Because we read or discuss it daily, our perceptions and attentiveness to medical professionalism have heightened, and our concept of a "professional" physician is very different than it was when we were undergraduates. Of the many definitions of professionalism, we find two to be particularly formative in our conception of medical professionalism. The first, from the Medical Professionalism Project, seems to address well the social or "external" view of medical professionalism. The first principle centers on patient welfare and altruistic dedication by the physician. The second principle values patient autonomy and patient involvement in medical decisions. The third principle, social justice, sees physicians as activists, working toward a more equitable distribution of health care (ABIM-F et al. 2002). The second definition, offered by some of our colleagues at the AMA, illustrates a perspective perhaps best articulated by physicians—a view from "inside" the profession. They write of medical professionalism as having three core elements: (1) moral commitment to the ethic of medical service (devotion to medical service and its values); (2) public profession of this ethic; and (3) professional advocacy for health care values in the context of other important and possibly competing values (Wynia et al. 1999). We see these three components as tightly woven elements necessary for best protecting sick and vulnerable persons in light of variable social and cultural attitudes.

Our study of those who have explored the charitable roots and fiduciary commitments of the medical profession, from its beginnings in the Hippocratic corpus to modern-day reflections, has shaped and enriched how we see ourselves as future doctors. To that end, in our callings to medicine, we are excited to put our largely theoretical encounters with professionalism to the test in our future work. It will likely not be an easy task. For example, medical residents are often underappreciated, underpaid, and work long hours. Pharmaceutical companies pay particular attention to them and opportunities will arise when medical professional conduct butts heads with industries and conflicts of interest arise that potentially promote harmful bias in patient care (Kassirer 2004).

Given the increasingly complex relationships between hospitals, insurance companies, academic medical centers, and the pharmaceutical industry, an education in the moral dimensions of medical professionalism, such as what we have received during our time with the AMA, will prove enduring and help us recognize more potential ethical dilemmas than we feel we would have otherwise. The physician role models we uphold emphasize the need to actively highlight these moral values in medicine, and we hope that we too will be able to identify and question professional behavior during our medical education with a critical eye, in situations large and small.

REFERENCES

American Board of Internal Medicine Foundation (ABIM-F), American College of Physicians (ACP), Academic Society for Internal Medicine Foundation (ASIM-F), and European Federation of Internal Medicine (EFIM). 2002. Medical professionalism in the new millennium: A physician charter. *Annals of Internal Medicine* 136(3): 243–46.

Kassirer, J. P. 2004. *On the Take: How Medicine's Complicity with Big Business Can Endanger Your Health.* New York: Oxford University Press.

Wynia, M. K., S. K. Latham, A. Kao, J. W. Berg, and L. Emmanuel. 1999. Medical professionalism in society. *New England Journal of Medicine* 341(21): 1612–16.

5

How Do You Tell Your First Patient He'll Die?

Andrew P. Jacques

How do you tell your first patient he'll die?

Medical school is filled with unspoken expectations. If I'm not worried I'll prove myself incompetent, I'm worried people will realize I don't always know what I'm talking about. I subconsciously expect that I'll pass tests and be able to answer an attending's questions about the mechanism of action of thiazide diuretics. If you had asked me before I started this year, I would have said that 90 percent of our job as physicians was to make people better and the other 10 percent was to help people to be comfortable as they passed away. This seemed a reasonable ratio to me, mostly healing and some comforting because, of course, everyone has to die. I never realized how much I expected to heal my first patient.

My first on-call experience was uneventful at best. I didn't admit a single patient and spent the majority of the night bored, all dressed up in royal blue scrubs sitting in the medical student lounge hoping to be paged. I slept fitfully in the tiny call room until my alarm woke me the next morning, a little disappointed no one had needed my "healing touch" throughout the night. So I was more than a little eager to get my hands dirty with this patient care stuff my second night in the hospital. It was around dinnertime. My senior resident instructed me to see a patient in the emergency room with suspected pancreatitis. I immediately rifled through the pages of my pocket-sized books to quickly read up on the topic in the elevator, and I organized the jumbled history and physical forms on my clipboard as I walked through the hallways. Ed*
complained of abdominal pain. An hour and a half later, my senior yanked me out of the room to run to the cafeteria before it closed. But

while Ed and I interacted, something magical happened. We introduced ourselves, I tried to make bad jokes at opportune moments, and he and I formed a physician-patient relationship. That night I told my fiancée, a fourth-year medical student, that if we looked hard enough in my seventy-seven-year-old patient, I was afraid we'd find something bad. My premonition was hauntingly accurate. His symptoms didn't fit the typical pattern of pancreatitis, and when we performed some diagnostic tests, they detected several liver lesions that were consistent with cancerous metastasis. I kept right on treating Ed, visiting him every morning, inquiring about his night's sleep, and pressing dutifully on his abdomen so I could detail my findings in daily progress notes. I talked with his wife, watched baseball with him on call, and heard stories of their grandson, a basketball player traveling Europe that summer. Ed wanted me to accompany him to have his liver masses biopsied, so I asked the nurses to page me when they performed the procedure. Ed and I talked while they took samples of his liver to examine under the microscope. Eleven days later we had to explain what all our testing meant. Ed had cancer and lots of it.

The cancer was so bad it had invaded his esophagus, next to his stomach, which explained Ed's recent loss of appetite and weight loss. He had the eight liver masses we'd first seen with ultrasound and confirmed with CT scan. The cancer had spread to his anterior mediastinum, lungs, and the lymph nodes around his celiac trunk, a major artery in the abdomen. The oncologist wrote "no hope of cure" in Ed's chart and wanted to discuss comfort care with his family.

I had been trying to prepare myself for a couple of days, knowing that the most likely result would be an unpleasant diagnosis. We walked in as a team: attending, senior resident, interns, and a frightened medical student. Ed paid close attention as our attending physician broke the terrible news. He seemed calm. As he did every day, he wanted to talk. He wanted to avoid the horrible truth of our presence with chit-chat, and we obliged him. Finally he looked directly at me and told me how lucky he had been to have me as his doctor. It was too much for me to handle, and I cried. Then, without breaking eye contact, he asked if people could survive this kind of cancer like he had survived prostate cancer. I had to tell him.

"I'm sorry, Ed," was all I could choke out. "Remember how we talked about cancer spreading?" I asked. No answer. I pointed to the places in his body the PET scan had shown as metastases and, choking back tears, I said, "It just is too many places. They can't do anything about it now."

While I was pointing to the cancerous growths, I couldn't help but feel that this was my last effort to heal Ed. If all our medical technology had failed, I reasoned, just maybe physical touch could produce a miracle no chemotherapy would furnish. As I touched Ed's pink skin I couldn't escape the truth of the cancer ravaging his body. I cried some more, and Ed told me it was okay and that I didn't need to be upset, something I thought was my job. We all talked to Ed as much as he wanted, and when I left that evening, part of me felt like I never wanted to return.

Ed and I talk about once a week now. I ate pizza with Ed and his wife the last time I stopped by. He tells me his pain is bad sometimes and that he wishes we could still talk every day. He gave me a watch he says he won't need anymore. I promise to pray for him and his family and to call again soon. I'm not sure who needs our conversations more, him or me.

*Permission sought and granted to use patient names. Surnames have been withheld to protect patient privacy.

6

Learning Japanese

W. Richard Boyte

"**D**octor, what nationality are you?"

Because minutes earlier Mrs. Hollingsworth had refused to speak to me, I was somewhat startled by her question. Her tone was not one of animosity or disrespect, but of sincere curiosity.

I had been leaning over to examine her motionless daughter, Sara. I straightened up to look at her. She sat at the opposite bedside dressed in old, loose-fitting military fatigues.

She repeated her question.

"American, I guess," I answered.

"No," she rejected my answer bluntly. "You're more than just 'American.' What's your race?"

I felt I should be more forthcoming. "Well, my father was from here . . . you know . . . from Mississippi. But my mother is Japanese," I explained.

"Ah ha!" she exclaimed in triumph, "I knew it." Her eyes brightened in excitement and her rigid posture began to relax.

"Does this bother you?" I asked cautiously.

"No. I just could tell. You don't look all white. Do you speak Japanese?"

"No. Never learned. My mother was afraid that I wouldn't speak English well."

"That's a real shame. I want to learn a lot of different languages. You know what I mean? Foreign tongues. I'm thinking about working at the UN as an interpreter."

"That's very interesting. Do you speak many foreign tongues now?"

"No. Just want to learn."

Attempting to take advantage of this unexpected opening, I quickly asked, "Could we move to the family conference room? We can discuss your daughter's situation in a more private setting." She exploded in anger, "No! Absolutely not! I will not let you kill my daughter! Is that understood? This conversation is over." With that, our first meeting came to an abrupt end.

I had arrived that Monday morning to take over the duties of attending physician in our pediatric intensive care unit. Sara Hollingsworth had been admitted to the PICU three days earlier. Her mother had been unable to arouse her from sleep that morning.

Upon their arrival to the trailer park home Sara shared with her mother, paramedics could not detect a pulse or effort to breathe from Sara. The teenager was rushed to the emergency department, where heroic measures restored a stable heart rhythm. From the outset, however, there was little hope for Sara to have a meaningful neurological recovery. The cause of her cardiopulmonary arrest would remain unclear.

Communicating with Mrs. Hollingsworth proved difficult. She was easily provoked to hostility and bitter suspicion. Short and small of frame, her demeanor and mannerisms nevertheless made her an intimidating figure. Her appearance was unkempt, and an overpowering odor of cigarette smoke clung to her oily black hair and her worn, dirty clothing. A neighbor informed a nurse that mental illness had long since caused her estrangement from friends and family.

Brain death was soon strongly suggested by Sara's physical examination. When Mrs. Hollingsworth was informed of plans for confirmatory tests on Sunday, she furiously insisted that none be performed. She demanded that all supportive measures, including mechanical ventilation, be continued. To do otherwise was, in her words, "cruel and inhumane." Attempts to discuss her concerns were met with scornful rage followed by impenetrable silence. My hopes that she might respond to me differently evaporated quickly.

The health care staff was holding several meetings each day over the difficult situation. By Wednesday, it was decided that confirmatory testing should be pursued even without Mrs. Hollingsworth's approval. Sara's prolonged suffering was frequently suggested as reason enough to proceed. Hospital administrators insisted that a court order be obtained. A judge granted an order to pursue testing on Thursday morning. It fell to me to inform Mrs. Hollingsworth.

She would not look at me as I approached Sara's bedside. Patients' beds in our PICU are separated from each other by nothing but a curtain. I knew that everyone within earshot would be paying close attention. My request to move to a more private setting was rebuffed by silence.

"Mrs. Hollingsworth, I have a court order to do testing. I will—"

"You will not," she said quietly.

"Actually, the decision has been made."

Instantly her faced became the tightly pinched result of unfiltered rage as she hurled a barrage of obscenities toward me. She moved in close to poke my chest with her index finger. I felt threatened, embarrassed, angry, and insulted.

"I will not let you perform your barbaric tests!"

"You have no choice."

"You cannot do this against my will!"

"I can. With the court order."

"I have never met anyone so cruel. You know I can't pay your bills. If that was a paying customer in that bed you wouldn't—"

At that moment my swirling emotions overcame all efforts to contain my temper. I shouted loudly, "Mrs. Hollingsworth! It is not about money! It is about your daughter! The tests are happening! You have no choice in the matter!"

Stunned by my sudden outburst, she stepped backward. In the uncomfortable silence that followed, she seemed to gather her thoughts. I waited nervously for her to speak.

"Wow," she said finally. "Your bedside manner really stinks."

The tests revealed no detectable brain function, and a diagnosis of brain death was declared. I would have to inform Mrs. Hollingsworth that all support measures would be withdrawn. I was congratulated by members of the health care team for bringing this difficult case to a resolution. But I felt no sense of satisfaction or triumph. After all, I had yelled at the mother of a dead girl.

I share with all physicians a heritage of professionalism carefully crafted over many years. Just as all cultural heritages do, medical professionalism has many languages associated with it. A good physician will learn to speak these languages with expertise. These are the tongues of compassion, of empathy, of understanding, of patience, of tolerance. Just as my cultural heritage does not endow me with an unlearned ability to speak Japanese, my heritage of medicine does not endow me with an unlearned ability to speak these languages of professionalism. Opportunities to learn these tongues must be recognized and embraced. Later that day, I reported the test results to Mrs. Hollingsworth. She appeared exhausted of spirit. She was allowing herself to begin grieving. I suddenly saw her for who she was, a frightened woman facing an uncertain future. Her daughter had been perhaps the only person in her life that was dear to her.

"Can I ask something? That is, can you do something for me?"

"I'll try," I replied.

"Can you give me just one more night with her?"

"Yes," I said.

She would not have the full night. Sara's heart stopped beating before sunrise. I returned to the hospital to give my condolences. Mrs. Hollingsworth had not left her daughter's side. She sat in quiet dignity as the nursing staff prepared Sara's remains for transfer to the morgue. I decided to sit with her. After a while, she was ready to leave.

"Thank you for giving me more time. I don't suppose you had to," she offered.

"I am just so sorry for your loss," I said.

She nodded and began to leave. Then she turned as if she suddenly recalled a pressing thought.

"You know, Doctor. You should really learn some Japanese."

"Mrs. Hollingsworth," I replied, "you're absolutely right."

7

In the Operating Room

Sandra McNeal

The senior orthopedics resident was performing a total knee reconstruction. I, the lone medical student, was watching from across the room. The residents were talking freely and joking with one another. The junior resident was enjoying the hands-on training provided by the senior. The circulating nurse was cheerful as usual. She was joking with the residents and teasing the scrub nurse. Everyone in the OR was enjoying the morning. When the resident reached a point in the surgery where the attending was required, Dr. Smith was called.

Dr. Smith burst into the room, hands dripping with water. He grabbed a towel from the scrub nurse and rushed over to the x-ray view box.

"Did you make the cut?" he demanded of the senior resident.

"No, we were waiting for you," the senior replied.

Dr. Smith stepped over to the table to view the resident's work.

"Did you measure before cutting?" he asked.

"We didn't cut anything. You told us to wait for you," said the senior.

"Good," said Dr. Smith as he finally put on his "space suit" and gloves.

Dr. Smith started measuring and preparing to cut the femur. While he was working, the residents updated him on one of his patients on the floor. The patient wanted to leave against medical advice, and Dr. Smith wanted the residents to convince the patient to stay. The residents explained that a fellow resident had gained the patient's trust and told the patient to leave. Upon hearing this, Dr. Smith roared, "Why did you let that f***er talk to my patient? From now on that f***er is not to go near any of my patients without one of you senior guys!"

55

The residents laughed uncomfortably and tried to explain that they had tried to convince the patient to stay. Dr. Smith demanded that the nurse page another resident to go upstairs and talk to the patient. Then he instructed the senior resident to cut the femur. He watched as the senior placed the saw against the bone. He then scolded the resident for placing the saw at an incorrect angle. After the bone was cut, Dr. Smith tried to place the prosthetic piece on the femur, but it did not fit. Dr. Smith flew into a rage.

"What the hell did you do?" he screamed at the senior resident.

The senior was upset and confused. He asked what he had done wrong.

Dr. Smith screamed, "It's just f***ed. It's just f***ed!" Dr. Smith acted as if he wanted to throw instruments across the room but thought better of it. He looked at the resident and said, "Don't you ever wonder why you never get a good fit? This always happens with you. I never have this problem with anyone else but you."

The resident again asked Dr. Smith to explain what went wrong and expressed a desire to learn from the mistake.

Dr. Smith screamed, "I don't even know what it is! It's just so f***ed! It's f***ed!"

The mood in the room was uncomfortably quiet. The circulating nurse was no longer cheerfully joking with the surgical nurse. The orthopedic company reps were busy searching for important messages on their digital organizers. No one spoke and no one made too many unnecessary movements. I wanted to leave, but was too afraid to move.

Dr. Smith was needed in another OR, so he took the saw and made some cuts to the bone. He told the resident to fit the prosthetic to the femur, then he left.

The senior resident asked people at the table if they had seen him do anything wrong. They had not seen anything wrong. The senior resident could not understand how he had made incorrect cuts when Dr. Smith had been guiding and observing him the whole time. In a display of emotional honesty unexpected from a surgical resident, the senior told the people at the table that Dr. Smith hurt his feelings. He said he always needs to drink after working with Dr. Smith.

The residents made more cuts to the bone and fit the prosthetic. While they waited for Dr. Smith to return, they talked about patients.

Their conversation was not as spirited as before, and it was limited to hospital-related topics. Dr. Smith returned in a surprisingly happy mood. He was cheerful and smiling when he entered the room. He even praised the senior's work. He and the residents finished the case without any outbursts of rage from Dr. Smith. Dr. Smith never apologized for his unprofessional behavior. He just acted as though it had never happened.

TEACHING PROFESSIONALISM

Teaching professionalism, as much as learning professionalism, requires reflection. Professional development is a lifelong dynamic process, and to teach effectively, educators must practice their craft. Therefore, without self-reflection, educators lose touch with the needs of their students and stagnate in their own professional development. The following essays are reflections by educators working to teach professionalism creatively and effectively.

8

Professionalism, Professional Autonomy, and the "Envelope of Knowledge"

David J. Doukas, M.D.

In a case conference on ethics with primary care residents, a senior family medicine resident presented the following case: A patient had come in requesting genetic testing in the primary care setting. A man in his thirties whose older brother had been diagnosed with Huntington's disease (HD) wanted to be tested for the genetic mutation that causes HD to see if he would have the same fate as his brother. The resident responded by offering him a referral to see a medical geneticist at the local major medical center several miles away.

The patient declined the referral for two reasons. He did not want to travel to see another doctor he did not know. Further, he wanted his own primary care doctor to perform the blood test, as they had known each other for a few years and he trusted his resident physician. Despite all attempts to persuade the patient to see the geneticist, the patient was adamant that he would not go to another physician for the test.

When this case was discussed during our case conference, the obvious question was, "What did you do?" The resident said that he performed the test, without consultation, and the results were negative. This ending might bring this story to a rapid close if not for several salient considerations. The resident was asked about prior medical school background coursework in human genetics and genetic counseling, which were quite scant. The resident's genetics experiences during residency were nil. The resident did note a lack of sufficient comfort level to perform the test and counseling, and he was contrite about not being at a level of proficiency expected of a genetics consultant.

At this point, a digression to consider the Accreditation Council on Graduate Medical Education (ACGME) General Competencies is appropriate (ACGME 1999). The General Competencies document was a bellwether for the current educational emphasis on professionalism. This document helps us address how we must teach and assess professionalism in residents, yet it cannot answer specific questions that arise in patient care. The "answer" is not always readily discernible. Both those advocating the resident's initial position and those opposing that position could claim a foundation in the General Competencies as a rationale for action.

From the provider's perspective, it is highly likely that the resident felt this therapy was "compassionate, appropriate, and effective for the treatment of health problems and the promotion of health" (ACGME 1999, Patient Care General Competency). Likewise, the resident was attempting to "demonstrate respect, compassion, and integrity, with a responsiveness to the needs of the patient that supercedes self-interest" (ACGME 1999, Professionalism General Competency). Nevertheless, the ACGME General Competencies also have expectations of what residents are to perform and what they are not to perform. Per the Interpersonal and Communication Skills Competency, the resident is expected to "work effectively with others as a member or leader of a health care team or other professional group" (ACGME 1999). Further, the resident is expected to "demonstrate a commitment to ethical principles pertaining to provision or withholding of clinical care, confidentiality of patient information, informed consent, and business practices" (ACGME 1999, Professionalism Competency). Likewise, the resident is expected to "advocate for quality patient care and assist patients in dealing with system complexities, and know how to partner with health care managers and health care providers to assess, coordinate, and improve health care" (ACGME 1999, System-Based Practice Competency).

With these many conflicting obligations, what is the resident to do? Is the resident exhibiting professionalism or not? On the resident's reflection, what seemed to be the "right" thing turned out not to feel so right. The pivotal role of the virtue of practical wisdom (also referred to as *phronesis*) is essential here, as it weighs the relative aspects of competing ethical considerations in caring for a patient. What may be the best action if the considerations are unopposed is very different than if the considerations are opposed by equally (or more) weighty considerations in the realm of professionalism. Two pivotal considerations drove the resident to act one way but later caused the resident to reassess the action and its possible consequences.

First, the resident succumbed to patient pressure to perform a service the resident did not feel comfortable performing. Yes, the test was straightforward in procedure (a blood draw) and would provide the patient with helpful knowledge (the good as defined by the patient). But the test is not straightforward in process—the person performing the test must be skilled in the task at hand. Whether it is in genetic testing, neurosurgery, or psychiatric counseling, the physician's expected level of competence needs to match that of a specialist who would perform the same task. While the risk of harm is always present in medicine, its likelihood rises exponentially when the practitioner's envelope of knowledge is pushed to, and through, the breaking point. The resident in this circumstance did not have the skills necessary to perform the requested service and as such should have referred the patient or declined the service.

Second, did the patient have a right to demand the test from the provider? If the provider has the necessary skill, such a request is plausible. However, we decline such requests when we do not have that knowledge. Further, despite the request, the provider is *not* required to provide a test or therapy merely because it is requested. This response is part of what is called professional autonomy (also known as integrity) in which the physician makes moral decisions of medical care—as they all ultimately are—that are in accord with the physician's own ability (based on knowledge and propriety of action as defined by that physician) to provide the service. Responding to patient demands with the refusal of such services requires tact and curbing the tide of hubris that lives within all physicians.

The essential aspect of this case is putting the patient into the hands of the provider that was required. No appeal to convenience here is pressing enough to warrant the resident's performing the test. The patient needed to be informed of the wisdom of gaining learned counseling from the geneticist and genetic counselor at the genetics clinic and to adequately process this information and make plans around it (if positive, to make future life plans, and if negative, to be counseled on possible survivor's guilt).

Did the resident act with professionalism? The resident deliberated most thoughtfully after the discussion of the case and realized how far over his head this case had gone. Realizing that one has gone outside one's knowledge area and created the potential for harm to the patient is growth of character that one hopes for in such cases. The real test is how the resident will respond the next time a patient asks for something outside the resident's envelope of knowledge. The need to train residents about the demands of being a physician requires the development of insight in the resident often not thought to be part and parcel of residency education (Doukas 2003; Doukas 2004). The explicit development of character needs to be made part of the language of ACGME education goals. It is the common denominator of how we expect residents to become physicians who are indeed professionals.

A fall from hubris can often result in a tough lesson in humility. Since the time of this case, I have frequently wondered how often physicians, whether they are residents or attending physicians, are "flying by the seat of their pants." An essential part of professionalism is clinical competence in what you know, but also knowing what you do not know. My concern in this case is the resident's acquiescence to the patient's demand and resistance to seeking appropriate counsel and consultation in a case that challenged the resident's knowledge and skill set. Some physicians have a hard time saying "I cannot" to themselves—even more than to their patients. As a teacher of physicians, I have often thought of how such a case is just the tip of many knowledge icebergs, whether it is regarding primary care practice, residency training, or physician autonomy. Such hubris should give us all great pause to consider this: How sure is any physician in his or her clinical care? I believe we would all do well to step back if we perceive our own envelope of knowledge straining while in the service of our patients.

REFERENCES

Accreditation Council for Graduate Medical Education (ACGME). 1999. Outcome Project, Competencies. Available: www.acgme.org/outcome/comp/compHome.asp. See also: www.bioethics.upenn.edu/faculty/doukas/classmodproj.html.

Doukas, D. J. 2003. Where is the virtue in professionalism? *Cambridge Quarterly of Healthcare Ethics* 12(2): 147–54.

———. 2004. Returning to professionalism: the re-emergence of medicine's art. *American Journal of Bioethics* 4: 18–19.

9

Developing Professional Skills

Mark G. Brennan

The universal recognition that education in medical ethics and professionalism should be a core component in the formation of physicians owes much to the pioneering and sustained efforts of clinical educators and bioethicists in the United States. Much of the current lively international debate regarding professionalism (Jotkowitz and Glick 2004) also originated in North America, where, for example, a major collaborative project on the subject resulted in the publication of a new charter (ABIM-F et al. 2002). In the United Kingdom, where progress had tended to be slower in these areas, the General Medical Council has encouraged the teaching of medical ethics and professionalism in its recommendations for undergraduate medical education (ABIM-F et al. 2002), and more recently in recommendations for postregistration training. Many British medical school curricula and postgraduate training programs now feature a professionalism component that is both clearly identifiable and assessable. My experience as a clinical educator in the United Kingdom suggests that there is a substantial group of doctors in training here (equivalent to residents in the United States) who missed out on these educational developments as medical students and are now keen to obtain further training in professionalism. These doctors are frequently working in the front line of medicine, where stress and a lack of experience, support, and training can lead to uncertainty about appropriate professional behavior and attitudes. As was once the case with medical ethics, it has sometimes been assumed that medical professionalism would be learned and understood through a process of osmosis, by observing what has been called the "well-disposed physician" in action. This assumption is obviously flawed as many undoubtedly good doctors in the UK still appear to be uncertain as to what constitutes professional behavior and good medical practice and seem to welcome structured guidance (General Medical Council 1999).

Between 2001 and 2005, the South Western Deanery in the UK (now known as the Severn Institute of the Severn and Wessex Deanery)—responsible for postgraduate medical education—provided a program titled Developing Professional Skills (DPS), which was made available to all doctors in training within the region. More than 250 participants took part in the program, which utilized attractive country house venues rather than hospital or university facilities. This included modules that covered generic aspects of professional life as a doctor, including time management, mentoring, teaching skills, medical ethics and law, and communication skills. Specialist training in the UK has been criticized for neglecting important aspects when preparing doctors for professional life in a career-grade post. Training by specialty can lead to a ghetto mentality that makes doctors fail to appreciate that many of the problems they face are generic rather than specialty-specific, as are the potential solutions. This mentality devalues the potential and actual collegiality of medicine, where the sharing of ideas, experiences, and information benefits all members of the medical family rather than only a tightly confined group.

A vital component of the DPS program was a two-day core module on professionalism run by the author and professor Colin Coles, which provided the opportunity for participants to reflect on a range of key topics. These included defining the meaning of professionalism; the challenge of being a professional in medicine twenty-four seven; leadership; the rewards, obligations, and privileges of being a doctor; practical sessions on time and stress management; and achieving or maintaining a work-life balance. An important aim was to encourage participants to identify and discuss what they perceive to be the positive aspects of being a doctor. The word *doctor* literally means teacher; good teachers are those who can inspire, guide, educate, lead, and bring out the best in others. Our participants usually had clear ideas about what makes a good or bad leader in medicine, but few of them had previously seen themselves as future leaders. We asked the doctors to present a case that described how they had dealt with a situation of uncertainty, where they had been required to exercise professional wisdom or discretion. This presentation was made in small groups with constructive feedback from fellow participants, facilitated by the course tutors; group confidentiality rules were agreed in advance of the presentations. It became clear that this small group session had a beneficial effect for many participants and a cathartic effect for some, especially where they were sharing an experience they found to be psychologically or emotionally traumatic. The therapeutic function observed in these sessions caused the course tutors to believe that—with the exception of a few specialties like family medicine, psychiatry, or anesthetics—opportunities for a nonjudgmental debrief outside this program were still worryingly rare for our participants.

The core module in the program received uniformly positive evaluations from participants, many of whom commented on the benefit of stepping out of the clinical environment—both literally and metaphorically—for two days. After what was called until 2005 the preregistration house officer (PRHO) year in Britain, and is now a two-year "Foundation Program" (equivalent to internship in the United States), doctors in the UK rarely have a formal opportunity to train or learn together with colleagues from other specialties and from primary and secondary care; this aspect of our course was rated particularly highly by participants. We found that our participants enjoyed discussing the nature and challenge of medical professionalism and by so doing had some of their enthusiasm for medicine restored. On the evidence presented by our participants, we believe that most doctors do their very best to remain professional—even when under extreme pressure on occasions. When they have failed to meet their own high standards, many participants acknowledged this and sought to improve their future performance. Learning from mistakes, admitting failure and error, and saying sorry should be a hallmark of all professionals, not just doctors. The responses of our participants indicate a real need for this type of postgraduate education in the UK and elsewhere, and we recommend the development of generic skills programs in those locations that have yet to do so. I have started to include elements of the DPS program for doctors training in the two-year Foundation Program in East Kent, and these have been well-received and evaluated highly by participants.

From a personal perspective, I have been greatly impressed by the altruism, honesty, and integrity displayed by many of the young doctors we have encountered in both the DPS and the Foundation Programs. They have willingly and generously shared experiences with one another in which they may believe themselves to have failed, appeared to expect negative criticism, and then have reacted with some surprise when instead their peers have offered them support, empathy, and affirmation. I have frequently heard it suggested that the actual practice of medicine dehumanizes the once idealistic medical student, and that initial optimism about a medical career is quickly replaced, following qualification, by cynicism. Our experience as medical educators is quite the opposite; we believe that many of the admirable values and virtues (e.g., seeking to care for others, wanting to make sick people better, aiming to work to the best of their ability, and selflessness) which informed the choice of a medical career were still intact in those we encountered in the program; true, a few of the values and ideals might be somewhat battered and bruised, but they have continued to motivate those we have met to be "good" doctors. The most heartwarming comments came from those who claimed that the DPS program—a limited intervention, as it was—had helped to restore some of their original enthusiasm for medicine and helped them to recognize that they had made the right career choice several years earlier. I have come to realize the benefits for doctors at all levels being able to take time out—literally to leave the ward, the theater, the consulting room, and the outpatient clinic—and spend time with colleagues from a range of specialties in a pleasant location away from the clinical setting, reflect, sometimes laugh and cry, and consider and discuss the purpose of medicine and their own place within the profession.

The author wishes to acknowledge with gratitude the work of his cotutor, Professor Colin Coles, and the DPS program administrator, Mrs. Barbara Burgess, without both of whose efforts the program would not have been the success it proved to be.

REFERENCES

American Board of Internal Medicine Foundation (ABIM-F), American College of Physicians (ACP), Academic Society for Internal Medicine Foundation (ASIM-F), and European Federation of Internal Medicine (EFIM). 2002. Medical professionalism in the new millennium: A physician charter. *Annals of Internal Medicine* 136(3): 243–46.

General Medical Council. 1999. *The Doctor as Teacher*. London: GMC.

Hatem, C. J. 2003. Teaching approaches that reflect and promote professionalism. *Academic Medicine* 78: 709–13.

Jotkowitz, A. B., and S. Glick. 2004. The professionalism movement—a more optimistic view. *The American Journal of Bioethics* 4(2): 45–46.

10

Failing at Teaching Professionalism

Amy Baernstein

I am motivated to teach professionalism when I witness its absence. My workplace, an urban Emergency Department, is a place where both patients and physicians are often frazzled. I see unprofessional behavior at times. These regrettable interactions, I think, are familiar to all: angry, intoxicated, shouting patient eventually gets under skin of overworked physician, who then growls back. Or worse.

Knowing that my second-year medical students will see behavior like this next year when they become clinical clerks, I ask them to consider the following scenario:

"Next year you will be working on the wards. Suppose you are watching your resident do a procedure on a patient. The resident has given the patient some local anesthesia, but it's not enough. The patient is clearly in pain, crying or even yelling, and asks the resident to stop and give him more pain medicine. The resident just says, 'I'm almost done, just let me finish' and keeps going. What should you do?"

My students give various sensible suggestions, but they are not the least engaged in this discussion. They clearly view my scenario as hypothetical, unrealistic. One of them says, "There are policies about giving adequate pain medicine. That wouldn't really happen." His tone of voice says, "Can we move on to something important?"

It is not news to anyone involved in the practice of medicine that this type of behavior happens, often. By naming "primacy of patient welfare" and "altruism" and the other principles of professionalism, we are trying to "educate" our trainees not to practice medicine like this. And I realize that I am not really asking my students, "What would you do if you saw this behavior?" I am asking them, "How can I make you not do things like this a few years from now?"

And who is this hypothetical resident, or practicing physician, ignoring the patient's anguish? How does that happen? Here's the stock answer: Empathetic, patient-centric human beings enter medical school. They are battered by an immense load of rote memorization, high-stakes exams, and competition among their peers. Residents working too many hours on too little sleep, and practicing physicians battered by managed care and other bureaucratic obstacles, are students' role models during their clinical training. Gallows humor and various dysfunctional coping mechanisms prevail, and voilà, the desensitized, dehumanized physician emerges.

There is some truth in this stock answer. Trying it on for size, I thought about my own medical training. How did I learn to be a professional? What forces and experiences created my professional behavior?

Students in their final year of medical school usually serve as "subinterns." During my subinternship, another student and I did the job of one intern, caring for hospitalized patients. Like interns, Adam and I were alone with patients at night. If a problem came up that we couldn't handle, we could call the supervising resident, who would advise us over the phone or, in extreme emergencies, come in to help us.

One night Adam and I faced a routine task, drawing a blood sample from a patient to check the level of an antibiotic. The blood had to be drawn at a specific time, which of course fell in the middle of the night. New to venipuncture, we went together. She was a "cross-cover" patient, meaning that someone else had primary responsibility for her care, and neither Adam nor I had the slightest knowledge of her or her medical problems. She was very, very old, and completely disoriented, whether from dementia or her acute illness or just the late hour, I don't know. We tried for veins in her arms, then hands, then feet, and failed. We decided that the best approach was to draw from her femoral vein, which runs under the crease where the leg meets the body. To get there we undid her diaper and folded her into a frog-leg position. Adam held her leg while I poked a long needle into her groin, looking for the vein.

It almost goes without saying that she started screaming. I couldn't find the vein, so Adam and I traded positions. He poked and poked while I leaned on her leg and held her wrists so she wouldn't grab at the syringe. I had my eyes fixed on the needle as Adam manipulated it, psychically willing it to finally hit the vein, but what I remember seeing most clearly was her thin gray pubic hair an inch away. I remember thinking "this must get done," and therefore I tuned out her screaming as best I could. I hate to admit that my exact thought was "be quiet, we're doing this whether you scream or not." And within an instant I had answered for myself something I had often wondered about but never understood: "This is how people are able to rape."

And so the blood was drawn and Adam and I went on about our other tasks that night. And neither of us is a monster; in fact we are both considered humanistic in our practice today. But there is no doubt that what I learned that night was how to ignore suffering and treat a human being like a piece of meat. Becoming a doctor, for me, meant learning to act in total opposition to the humanistic values we say we are trying to cultivate in our students.

I can easily critique "the system" that allowed this particular nightmare to unfold. First, Adam and I were inexperienced. We should have had someone to turn to who could draw the blood without torturing the patient. I don't believe we were either too arrogant or too cowardly to ask for help; we were told in subtle and not-so-subtle ways that calling our resident for help with "scut" was unacceptable. Furthermore, collaboration between nurses and doctors at that institution at that time was poor, and since nighttime blood draws were "doctor" jobs, we felt we could not appeal to the nursing staff for help. Finally, in retrospect, I question whether midnight blood draws were clinically appropriate for that patient.

However, even if this scenario could have been prevented, I believe the situation is universal: medical training inevitably requires trainees to treat a patient as less than a person. Some clinical situations require action that disregards the patient's immediate comfort, and at other times a patient's experience is too outrageous to be accessible to us, their physicians. My pre–medical school self would be appalled by my conduct that night, and yet I see it now as a necessary aspect of training. What is not necessary is the habit that some physicians develop in response to experiences like this: the habit of perceiving patients as nonpeople more than is absolutely necessary.

One reason our "discussions" of professionalism with our students fall so flat is that we tiptoe around certain topics. Our classroom conversations have much in common with the stories that doctors write for publication: despite some trying circumstance, the fundamentally noble patient teaches the now humbled doctor an important lesson. And certainly these events occur in real-life medical practice. But other moments of high drama occur because both patients and doctors are human, in a bad way. These are the stories that are rarely talked about in public. Students without clinical experience are deeply offended by these stories. Doctors in practice know better than to put them in writing. But failing to acknowledge this part of medical reality contributes to our problems in "educating for professionalism," namely that our exhortations about proper behavior have a preachy tone.

I think we might make better inroads with our students by admitting that both doctors and patients can be unpleasant, dishonest, and infuriating. Furthermore, the practice of medicine can put doctors and patients together under the worst possible circumstances. If we were more willing to portray the flaws of doctors, patients, and the practice of medicine itself, and more prepared to describe the unspeakable events that can happen even when we try our best, I think our students might be able to use such events to advance their professionalism rather than destroy it.

My second-year students say they can't imagine feeling angry toward a patient. They are likely to have even less acceptable feelings soon, and when they do, I would like to help them behave humanely even when they don't feel that way. I believe more honesty about our less-than-noble thoughts and actions would help achieve this goal. If we have the courage to tell our real stories, the ones that are not appropriate for prime time, the ones that are not our proudest moments, perhaps our students will learn to respond to similar situations with behavior we can applaud.

I would like to thank Adam Cifu, M.D., for allowing me to share this story, and I would like to ask forgiveness from the patient described.

11

"On Professionalism" Course

Denise Gibson

"On Professionalism: Promoting Professionalism in an Unprofessional World" was first offered as a four-week interdisciplinary course at Northeastern Ohio Universities College of Medicine spring term 2003. This was an elective course in the Human Values in Medicine program (referred to by students in their writing as HVM), a component of the Department of Behavioral Sciences. Fourth-year medical students met for eight hours a week for four weeks and considered different ideological perspectives on professionalism with various class lectures and reading assignments. Active class discussion was an expectation of all seven students who enrolled, and a short reaction paper was required after each class.

Excerpts from the seven students' reaction papers follow. As the director for the course, the experience of teaching medical professionalism in the classroom was rewarding, enlightening, and invigorating. Throughout the course but especially at the end, students gave feedback about the course and offered recommendations for future course offerings.

This HVM course surprised me in many ways. It made me think about issues that most medical students rarely consider. And even if I have dealt with similar issues, I don't think they had the same meaning as they do now. The common sentiment of the group throughout the four weeks was that this is a class that all the students could really benefit from. (A.A.)

The final discussion on residency training and patient views was a great way to wrap up all of the discussions for the last class meeting. The patients made very good comments about issues I had not even considered. (A.A.)

When Dr. Hafferty passed out the article in class entitled, "Do Clinical Clerks Suffer Ethical Erosion?" I was not surprised at the numbers and percentages listed in the abstract (i.e., 62% reported that they suffered some form of ethical erosion). The world of medicine that we're taught to believe in during the first two years of medical school is a closed, ideal medical world . . . sort of a medical utopia or Shangri-la. I think almost every student who makes the transgression from basic sciences to clinical clerkships experiences a form of disillusionment when on the wards. The reality of the wards is like any other workplace—the residents, nurses and attendings are tired, stressed and in such adverse situations, their behavior is not always the most ethical. (A.F.)

When you mentioned that we could write about how our views on professionalism have changed since beginning this HVM course, at first I thought, well, my views don't feel they've changed that much—in the sense that I haven't had any profound epiphanies about the concept of professionalism. But, reflecting about it, I realize that I have a better sense of the concept of professionalism. I am definitely more cognizant of its importance and the integral role it plays for us as future physicians. I have a better idea of how to define professionalism—a concept that has always been elusive when trying to make it concrete. . . . I have learned of the role of professionalism in public health policy and from a social point of view. I have learned about the history of professionalism. All of these different aspects have rooted the concept and make it multi-dimensional. I believe that the concept should take root in medical school and one should expect to spend a lifetime trying to attain and become that ideal professional. It should be considered the pinnacle marking of a successful physician. (A.F.)

As we approach graduation, many of us are very apprehensive about having enough knowledge and skills to be good physicians. What this HVM has done for me, at least, is change my focus . . . being a good doctor isn't just about mastering the necessary skills and abundant facts . . . it's about being compassionate, altruistic, having the strength to put aside one's personal views and see through the eyes of the patient. It's about duty and excellence and always challenging oneself to keep up with those ideals. Most importantly, it's about being cognizant that one must uphold a concept of professionalism and make it a part of one's moral fiber. You have to live it to be it. (A.F.)

Looking back on the last 3 1/2 weeks, I am quite happy with the decision I made to take the "On Professionalism" HVM. In accordance with the other students who took this class, I strongly believe that every fourth-year student should be required to take this course prior to graduation. During medical school, we often heard the term "professionalism" being used, but never really had a full grasp on what the term signified. With residency a few months away, I feel that now more than ever, we need to know what it really means and why it has been such an important topic in medicine. . . . To me, professionalism is a set of qualities and traits that one can possess, including integrity, altruism, knowledge, compassion, dedication, and a passion for life-long learning. As a physician, these are qualities that we must all strive to achieve. I feel it is more ideal because, for example, one will never know everything there is to know about medicine (or their own specialty) or be able to treat all patients equally without the interference of personal bias. Having gone through this class has made me really look at my own belief system and how I plan on handling the challenges of being a physician in the upcoming years. (M.G.)

The discussion on the article pertaining to the Medical School Objectives Project (MSOP)[1] made me think about these issues on a broader spectrum. I began to wonder why these principles are not being enforced or even employed in other health-related fields. Other health care–related professionals such as managed care and pharmaceutical companies seem to be exempted from the same edicts that are demanded and expected from physicians. Why should we be the only group subjected to such intense scrutiny and liability to remain professional? . . . It is difficult for physicians or medical students to be altruistic, knowledgeable, skillful, and dutiful when at every turn they are faced with a direct and opposing force from within the system. . . . The road is difficult for physicians when there are so many obstacles to overcome and it seems to be an act of futility unless there is redirection of *all* parts of the system in one collaborative approach to professionalism. (T.K.)

Ethics is a component of professionalism and many times is used as a synonym. I do not really believe this is the proper use of the term. While ethics is a significant component of professionalism, it should not be mistaken for all of it. Clearly, the American Board of Internal Medicine has outlined four other components in which to dissect this term of professionalism.[2] Altruism, knowledge, skill and duty may not be the best way to define professionalism but it is the beginning of our attempt to define the concept that means different things to so many people. (T.K.)

The reading assignment [P. Starr, *The Social Transformation of American Medicine*, Chapter 3, The Consolidation of Professional Authority,

1850–1930][3] was a great perspective from an outsider's viewpoint on the development of organized medicine. It chronicled the very beginning of organized medicine and detailed the struggles of allopathic medicine in defining itself. I learned that many of the other branches of healthcare grappled with establishing their identity as well as respect with the community. It seems as though allopathic medicine was able to win respect through standardization of education as well as the code of ethics. This code of ethics was the early development of some components of our modern-day interpretation of what we believe is professionalism.

I found the majority of the early code of ethics focused on bringing respect and controlling the perception of medicine. This must have been essential because the profession was still proving itself to the public. It directed physicians to respect the profession as well as each other in an effort to show patients that medicine was truly an honorable career. This in turn brought patients back to allopathic physicians over other healthcare providers as a now unified profession commanded the respect it so fervently strove for. (T.K.)

My perspective on professionalism has broadened significantly since the beginning of this elective. I was wondering what our group would be able to discuss and learn over a span of 32 hours. I must admit that I was pleasantly surprised with the content of the course as well as the thought-provoking discussions we shared. The progression of the topics was also very well thought out and immensely informative.

I think that there is a widely accepted misconception that this idea of professionalism is strictly unique to our school. . . . This class seems to be sorely misplaced in the curriculum and should not be an elective at the end of medical school but should rather be placed in the first grading period of the first year. Many times by senior year there is a strongly ingrained disdain for yet another mention of "professionalism." Too many students think that they already know what it is and they in truth do not. (T.K.)

Hafferty's chapter "In Search of a Lost Cord"[4] is correct when he says that professionalism needs to be readdressed and prioritized. A large part of what medical students learn about professionalism and professional behavior is learned through the "hidden" or informal curriculum. I actually believe that this is true in professional schools overall. . . . Mentoring is so pivotal. Mentoring others, thereby becoming teachers of the informal curriculum, is an extremely important aspect of being a professional.

Influences such as societal expectations of physicians, increased responsibilities, and managed care expectations have played a large part in the changing face of medicine. Medical schools, understandably but not excusably, have tried to answer these expectations at the expense of professionalism values. (J.L.)

Professionalism truly means caring for/relating to/interacting with people whose opinions or behaviors differ from your own—because, in doing so, you may be enlightened about others' points of view and you may be able to enlighten them too.

At our initial meeting, we all tried to identify aspects of professionalism—what does it include, what does it mean to us, how do we try to ensure its presence in our daily patient interactions? We also found that most of us took this elective with an interest in self-improvement and discussion of professionalism issues. Our class sessions were challenging, revealing, and fun! As I reflect on this class, I know that we haven't arrived at any "grand conclusions," we haven't created a professionalism curriculum, we haven't designed assessment tools, we haven't arrived at the final answer to the question, *"What is professionalism?"* This is not a bad thing! As we've mentioned in class, it is difficult for us to discuss a nebulous concept like professionalism. We aren't used to this, and we feel uncomfortable with the unmeasurable nature of this concept. However, I think it is not only acceptable but *preferable* that we didn't try to focus too much on capturing or quantifying what professionalism is. It forced us to talk about, reflect upon, and become more comfortable with this vague but important concept. Ideally, we will continue to do this on our own as we encounter professionalism issues in our future. . . . I think this course has given all of us the tools for self-reflection and analysis in order to become better, more professional physicians. That, in the end, is the most beneficial part of this entire experience. Thanks for this wonderfully creative, constructive, and challenging four weeks! (J.L.)

What I will take away from this course is that ethical behavior is part of professionalism. Putting the patient first is an obligation, one that has been part of being a physician in American since 1847 (i.e., with the first AMA guidelines).[5] (E.R.)

In this world of professionalism and in an effort to project an image of prestige, we as physicians sometimes miss the whole point—we are called to action for our patients. I can get wrapped up in congratulating myself on my ability to escape the "physician perspective" and the air of dignity at all costs that I sometimes forget that the patient is why I am here. I find myself trying to detach from the arrogance associated with being a physician. I have been in situations that would have called for a touch of humanism but I was too afraid to do so for fear of sacrificing my dignity or respect as a future physician. Physicians perform physical exams and remove articles of clothing and don't return them because the nurse will do it. I told myself I never want to get to the point where I believe I am more important than the patients I care for. When I remove a patient's socks, I place them back on their feet because I am not above that. It is not compromising my professionalism by doing humane things for patients. (M.R.)

During this course there have been some enlightening and informative discussions about what it means to be professional. At the beginning of the course I had a vague sense that professionalism was a standard of behavior or code of ethics that is defined by people of a particular occupation. Similar to most people's ideas, I thought professionalism is implied by your manner of dress, interactions with people, and authoritative status in society. The standards that signify professionalism could be applied to members of any occupation. Yet this course has helped me redefine my views and attitudes toward professionalism from the perspective of a physician. I like to think that professionalism is an ideal that I can strive to achieve—ideals such as altruism, integrity, honor, excellence, duty and commitment. I realize this is a lifelong process and I must be cognizant of my professionalism and willing to evaluate and redefine my concepts of professionalism as I become more knowledgeable. It was helpful to have a forum to discuss ideas and experiences with professionalism. (M.R.)

The students' journal entries speak volumes about the course, its curriculum, and the process each experienced by having taken an elective in medical professionalism. For me, student feedback about the course offered insight about what students understood regarding the concept of professionalism coming into the course and what they *need* to understand as they graduate from medical school. Their honesty about how professionalism is taught (or not) is compelling because they point out how the concept needs to be taught in a meaningful way throughout medical education. I hope the words of my students will assist other faculty members in medical education who teach courses in professionalism or who are compiling courses in professionalism to continue the valuable lessons in educating medical students to become professional physicians.

I end this article with the words of one particularly literate student in the course who was inspired to write a poem about what professionalism means to her:

PROFESSIONALISM

Putting the patient's care/wishes/needs first

Remember that "the patient is why I'm here"

Overcoming obstacles to appropriate behavior (stress, pressure, time constraints, personal issues, patient load)

Finding a way to care for patients when you don't agree with their views/ideas/values

Ethical treatment of patients and ethical personal behavior, even getting ethics consultations if necessary

Self-awareness of knowledge base, knowledge gaps, biases, and values—and how these impact patients

Stretching personal limits to best serve your patients

Integrity, truth, and honesty in dealing with patients and their friends/family members

Openness and respect for patients/peers/others

Needing to take care of yourself so that you may better treat your patients

Attempting to put yourself in the patient's shoes so you may better understand them

Lifelong learning and a commitment to self-improvement (for yourself and ultimately for your patients)

Intelligence, with the understanding that intelligence alone does not equal professionalism

Seeking peers with similar professionalism values

Mentoring other medical and allied professionals in order to foster professionalism in future colleagues

NOTES

The author wishes to give special acknowledgment to the seven students in the course who contributed significantly to this article. Their specific contributions are noted in the article by the initials of their name: Amol Arora, M.D., Aysha Farooqi, M.D., Monica Gogate, M.D., Timothy Ko, M.D., Jeanne Lackamp, M.D., Erin Rinto, M.D., and Mesie Rogers, M.D.

1. The Medical School Objectives Writing Group. 1999. "Learning objectives for medical school education—Guidelines for medical schools: Report I of the Medical School Objectives project." *Academic Medicine* 74(1): 1–13.

2. Project of the ABIM Foundation. ACP-ASIM Foundation and European Foundation of Internal Medicine. 2002. "Medical professionalism in the new millennium: A physician charter." *Annals of Internal Medicine* 136(3): 243–46.

3. P. Starr, 1982. *The Social Transformation of American Medicine: The Rise of a Sovereign Profession and the Making of a Vast Industry.* New York: Basic Books.

4. F. W. Hafferty, 2000. "In search of a lost cord: Professionalism and medical education's hidden curriculum. In *Educating for Professionalism: Creating a Culture of Humanism in Medical Education.* Edited by D. Wear and J. Bickel. Iowa City: University of Iowa Press.

5. American Medical Association. 1867. *Code of Medical Ethics/Adopted by the American Medical Association.* New York: William Wood & Company.

PERSONAL AND PROFESSIONAL IDENTITY CONFLICT

Physicians are people first. Most of the time professional and personal values integrate seamlessly, but not always. Over their careers, all professionals encounter situations that put their personal identity in conflict with their professional identity. Professional values and skills dictate how professionals as individuals deal with these tensions and maintain professional dignity and respect for their patients. The reflections in the following section demonstrate professionals' capacity to overcome personal value conflicts while maintaining their integrity as people and physicians.

12

Veiling the Scrubs

Mona Ahmed

Write the bad things that happen to you on sand. Write the good things that happen to you on marble.

Arabic proverb

The summer before starting medical school, I read the book *Making of a Surgeon* by William Nolen. It was a narrative account of a surgeon's internship years that recalled the astonishing procedures and techniques he was able to master during his residency. This inspiring novel captured the gleam of how remarkable it is to be able to perform surgery. The technique, confidence, creativity, quick decision-making, and responsibility the story revealed inspired me to dream of becoming a surgeon myself. I wanted to save lives and solve problems. William Nolen became my hero. The back cover of the book showed a photograph of him, and I would look at his hands. Few people can do what he does, and few people have miraculous hands like his. I wanted miraculous hands, too. I wanted to be like William Nolen.

At the beginning of my freshman year, I sought the opportunity to observe surgery. I decided to go for a fancy procedure—cleft palate reconstruction on an infant. I was going to watch somebody perform a miracle because I wanted to learn how to perform them. One thing, however, had slipped my mind.

Scrubs.

Surgeons wear scrubs.

Everybody in the OR wears scrubs.

In fact, everybody on the second floor of our hospital wears scrubs.

It logically followed, then, that I too had to wear scrubs. This, however, posed a peculiar problem.

I am a Muslim woman who wears the Islamic veil. According to Islamic tradition, Muslim women are to dress modestly in front of men they are not related to. Modest Islamic garb includes long sleeves up to the wrists, long pants or skirts that reach the ankles, and a veil that covers the head, the neck, and the ears. I wrap my head in colorful and patterned veils that reveal only my face.

How was I going to wear scrubs?

I asked the receptionist of the second-floor surgical unit. She did not have an answer for me. Instead she asked me a question . . . with her eyes. "Why do you have to be so difficult?"

"Ma'am, I'm supposed to keep my head and neck covered. What do I do?"

"You wear a cap with scrubs."

"What about my neck?"

"I'll give you towels."

Towels for my neck? I wondered if we were speaking the same language.

She ended the conversation by telling me the changing rooms were on my right. I followed a kind lady in who realized I was new to this scene and directed me to the scrubs and the caps. My plan was to wear two caps over my head. (Ideally, that would have covered my ears, but I later on realized that my golden studs were blatantly visible.) Then I would run over to the receptionist's desk and drape towels over my neck. My arms would be exposed, yet my priority remained my head. After all, the first thing people would see when they looked at me would be my head.

My head. That's exactly what everybody saw—my head. I had to pass through the surgical waiting area, on the other side of the female changing rooms, amidst the scrubbed surgical staff on my way to the reception desk. Men and women were everywhere, but I saw only the men. Those men saw my hair through the transparent surgical caps. They saw my earrings, they saw my neck, and they saw my bare arms. I felt like I was in public without a skirt on. The last time any man besides my father had seen this sacred and protected view of me was when I was twelve years old. I stood there as an embarrassed twenty-two-year-old woman. Everything dear to me was exposed to men—not just to strangers but to male students and attendings who had seen me in my sacred veil at school. I frantically searched for the reception desk. "Can I have the towels now?" By this time vulnerability was overwhelming my existence. I was defenseless without my veil. The lady shouted back at me. "Do you need them right now?" I responded like a shocked, silent puppy. My head was low, my eyes glued to the floor. Was I a destitute dog waiting for somebody to show mercy on me by throwing me a bone to stay alive? Human beings should be treated with dignity. I was not an animal, nor was I a child. Ten minutes seemed like ten hours, after which the woman gave me the towels. I had a blue fluffy cap, resembling a sheep, on my head and two matching tea towels draped around my neck. I was ready to watch surgery.

The surgeon came and took the baby to the OR. Inside the OR, I stood in the corner, by the telephone, for three hours. The cold in the OR sent chills down my spine and gave me goose bumps. It was a constant reminder of my lack of clothing. I was not allowed to enter the sterile field and from my corner it was difficult to get a view of the little baby's wide-open mouth from a distance amidst the crowd around the table. I politely excused myself from the OR and rushed back to change into my long sleeves and silky black veil. All that for nothing.

After this first disappointing experience of watching surgery, I decided I never wanted to wear scrubs again. That would make a three-month surgery clerkship and a career as a surgeon extremely difficult. We enter medical school with dreams, aspirations, energy, and hope, and it is painful to see them quickly crushed. I had to let go of something, and I was definitely keeping my veil, so William Nolen had to go.

Luckily, I go to a Jesuit medical school. We have a ministry center operated solely for the spiritual and social assistance of the students. Even more luckily, I had a physician mentor who asked me about my experience in the OR and helped me realize that the situation could be resolved. My dreams and my confidence had been shaken, but my mentor and a ministry staff member lifted my spirits. They empowered me and encouraged me to stick to my principles to resolve my issue. I was directed to the surgical administrative nurse, who was friendly, sympathetic, and very helpful.

Somewhere, sometime, a genius invented the "bearded man's cap." It makes me look like Lawrence of Arabia, but it keeps my head, ears, and neck perfectly covered. Now I wear two scrub shirts, one backward and one forward to keep my chest covered. When I do not need to scrub, I wear a scrub jacket to cover my arms. So far, this technique has worked in my experiences observing in the labor rooms. When I start my surgery clerkship in two years, I know there will be eyes on my head as I wear my cap and appear dressed differently. However, I appear dressed differently even when I am not in the OR. If I am destined to have unwanted glares, those eyes can see me covered rather than exposed.

In the 1960s, my mother's struggle as a medical student was her presence as a woman in a world of medicine dominated by men. In 2005, my struggle is to balance religious freedom in the world of medicine. I am definitely not the first Muslim veiled woman to have come across this problem. I am sure there are Muslim veiled women out there who work in surgical fields. Maybe few are seen because there are few of them. I was forced to act like a pioneer because I was one of the first Muslim veiled students at my school, and I hope I have carved a pathway to make life easier for others treading the path after me. Scrubs should not be the reason why people like me would choose to be invisible in surgical fields. If I still decide on pursuing a surgical specialty as my career, I can. While adorning my head with the "bearded man's cap" in place of the veil, I can still have miraculous hands. I can still perform miracles. I can still be like William Nolen.

13

Family Physician

Kathy Stepien

Eyebrows raise in curious surprise. I'm not on his schedule. He does not expect to see me in the busy clinic hallway. I turn over the pamphlet entitled "miscarriage" to answer his unspoken question. Sadness instantly crosses his face. Without hesitation, he gives me a full frontal, two-armed, stethoscope-in-the-way hug.

He will read my chart later to learn about the spotting at ten weeks. The cessation of my nausea and fatigue. The report from his colleague saying no fetal heartbeat was found on pelvic ultrasound. He will see me in his office in a few days when the bleeding has not stopped, and he will take time away from his own family to perform the D&C.

Neither knows the events of the miscarriage that will unfold, but we both know he will be there to help if he can. I break our silent exchange, say thanks, and move on. He has other patients waiting for him. I have tears to cry in private. The miscarriage proceeds but the healing begins.

14

Not of Our Choosing

Bonnie Salomon, M.D.

When I was a little girl, my father used to tell me, "You can choose your friends, but you can't choose your relatives." It was his lesson in practicality and reality, in acceptance, and understanding the difference between choice and circumstance. As an emergency physician, sometimes that saying comes back to me, but in a variation to suit my position: "You can choose your practice, but you can't choose your patients." As any emergency physician can attest, our patients are whoever walks in the door or arrives by ambulance. I have absolutely no choice over whom I treat, making the practice free of financial bias, socioeconomic concerns, or any latent prejudices. It is an entirely democratic way of being a doctor: we take care of everyone, regardless of any consideration. Unfortunately, not everyone who walks in the door is pleasant, grateful, cooperative, or even sober. That aspect of the job is well-known to anyone who's done a shift in an emergency department. But what of a truly hateful patient, a morally despicable patient, the kind of person who is a threat to me and to society? Taking care of such patients might be a moral hazard. These kinds of patients test my professionalism as well as my compassion.

Take the case of the neo-Nazi. It was New Year's Eve at Cook County Hospital in Chicago. I was on my trauma rotation as an emergency medicine resident from Northwestern. Apparently, the highlight of the evening for any hooligan is to shoot his gun into the night air at the stroke of midnight. We had multiple patients arrive as the new year rolled in—gunshots to various extremities as well as some serious chest and abdominal injuries. I was low man on the totem pole that night, only a second-year resident, so I was given the relatively "minor" gunshot wounds.

My patient was a young man with short black hair who presented with a gunshot wound to his foot and abdomen. As the trauma team took off his clothes, I couldn't help but see a large swastika tattooed on his chest. I paused, if just for a second. During a trauma resuscitation, the infamous "golden hour" where time is critical, there is no time for personal reflection, and certainly no place for assessing the morality of your patient. It is a time for action, for the placement of IV lines, X-rays, catheters, etc. It is a time when all your energies should be focused on the patient on the gurney.

So while I glanced at the swastika, the doctor part of my brain did what it was taught to do. The white lab coat, however, does not erase all personal memories or feelings. Let me elaborate. My parents are Holocaust survivors. They survived years of Nazi brutality in various death camps. I grew up with an intimate knowledge of how the Nazis tortured and killed my grandparents, aunts, uncles, and cousins. The swastika is a particularly insidious symbol to me. In some ways, it has always evoked some fear, since it is a symbol of a group that believes my family should all be murdered.

So there I was, a second-generation Jewish-American, treating a neo-Nazi at Cook County Hospital. His system of beliefs called for my death. Yet there I was, working hard to save his life. Of course, I found him morally repugnant, and I must admit I was somewhat fearful. The gist of the situation was this: I was his doctor, and he was my patient.

The physician-poet Dannie Abse wrote a striking poem about a similar situation (caring for a hateful, bigoted patient) in "Case History":

> "Most Welshmen are worthless,
> an inferior breed, doctor."
> He did not know I was Welsh.
> Then he praised the architects
> Of the German death-camps—
> Did not know I was a Jew.
>
> (Abse 1995)

However repugnant this patient is to Abse, he treats him in a professional manner. Abse goes to the clinic's pharmacy, when he finds all sorts of poisons. While he emotionally considers such dastardly medicine, as a professional he never harms this horrible man. Abse writes:

> Yet I prescribed for him
> As if he were my brother.
>
> (Abse 1995)

Abse's poem echoes quite a bit for me, having cared for many hateful patients, the kind of person you'd avoid in any other social setting. The practice of medicine, while social, is unlike other encounters. Patients expect a physician to treat them in a professional way, free of prejudice, free of disdain. The model for this is a *fiduciary* relationship—an ethical imperative that the physician "owes undivided loyalty to those served and must work for their benefit" (Jonsen, Siegler, and Winslade 1998, 157).

How difficult it is in the real world to owe "undivided loyalty" to a bigoted, sociopathic patient. How difficult it is to work for the benefit of an individual who abhors you, who wishes harm to you and your family, who cannot stand other people like you. Yes, it is extremely difficult, but that is what a physician can and must do on a daily basis. Imagine the state of affairs if doctors only treated patients of their choosing, or patients they found pleasant and cooperative. While that world might sound appealing to physicians, I suspect most of us, in our heart of hearts, recognize how wrong it would be. When a young man or woman chooses to become a physician, he or she also chooses (perhaps unknowingly) to care for patients who may be difficult, abhorrent, or even dangerous. Physicians must acknowledge these painful issues, but at the same time they must acknowledge they are a critical aspect of our chosen profession. We cannot take only the good, neglect the bad, and ignore the rest. The physician-philosopher Maimonides put all this in perspective in his Oath. For me, it is a line full of wisdom and humanity, a creed that all physicians should live by:

> In the sufferer, let me see only the human being.

There it is—a simple line, yet profound and exceedingly relevant. No matter how despicable, unpleasant, or hateful that sufferer is, let me see only the human being. If I can do that, I can live up to the standards of my profession, and I can be a true physician.

REFERENCES

Abse, D. 1995. "Case history." In *On Doctoring*. Edited by R. Reynolds and J. Stone. New York: Simon and Schuster.

Jonsen, A. R., M. Siegler, and W. J. Winslade. 1998. *Clinical Ethics: A Practical Approach to Decision Making in Clinical Medicine.* 4th ed. New York: McGraw-Hill.

THE PATIENT'S VOICE

The final essay reminds us that the ultimate goal of teaching and learning professionalism, and acting professionally, is to improve the patient's experience. Everything a physician does, even personal enrichment, derives its professional value from its impact on patients. Professional development and reflection are key factors in the mission of medicine—to ease suffering—and thus the following patient perspective is invaluable.

15

A Patient Reflects . . .

Thomas Schindler

Nothing directs your attention to quality health care quite like being hit by a truck. When you finally recover your senses—weeks after the accident—you find yourself in a hospital with no idea how you got there or how long you'll be there. You have tubes protruding from your body, and you are dependent on the staff to bring you whatever you need. When you want to walk, you have to go to therapy. You can't take a shower by yourself. You even have to let someone at the desk "buzz you out" to leave the floor. Being so completely dependent makes you appreciate quality, "professional" health care like never before. It makes you appreciate professionalism in those who provide that care. I have such new appreciation; I was the driver of a car hit by a semi, and I survived to share these reflections.

Before my accident I did not consider myself a stranger to the medical profession. Both my parents had suffered serious illness and both had endured lengthy hospitalizations. Thirty years ago I worked as a night administrator at a large community hospital in Chicago and considered myself a member of the "team." In recent years I had undergone physical therapy for a knee injury and ended up with a total knee replacement. The truck, however, made all these earlier encounters with the medical profession seem insignificant by comparison. Suddenly, I was dependent and the focus of care, and I cared about that care in a way I never had before.

The invitation to share my reflections on professionalism also stems from an ongoing conversation with one of the editors of this collection of essays. For several years she and I have tossed around ideas about what constitutes professionalism in various fields. I used to have difficulty defining professionalism; now I feel fairly certain that I know it when I see it.

What makes someone a "pro" in his or her field? An athlete, a brick-layer, a mechanic, a plumber is a pro when someone pays for his or her services. Yet we use "professional" in another sense, too. The pro is so good at what he or she does, and does it in such a pleasing way, that we recommend him or her to others without being asked. "You need a brake job? I've got a shop that's fantastic. They'll do your brakes the same day and guarantee their work for a full year. Who else will give a guarantee like that on brakes? And they don't charge an arm and a leg, either."

When someone doesn't measure up to our admittedly subjective standards, we have no qualms about telling others that as well. "You need brakes? Stay away from _____. They have great prices and work fast, but you'll need new brakes again in just two months. And they are really rude."

In preparing to write this essay, I paid particular attention to the unsolicited observations of friends and family as to what they liked or disliked about their medical providers. In my attempt to synthesize these comments and integrate them with my own ideas, I've come up with certain characteristics of medical providers that I consider at least somewhat indicative of professionalism in the medical field.

So what qualities do we appreciate in our doctors or nurses or therapists? What makes them "professional" in our eyes? What makes us tell others how good these professionals are? What makes us pass along their names and phone numbers? The following qualities are not in any particular order. Some will be more important than others according to the perception of the evaluator, the type and seriousness of the condition being treated, and the personal values of each individual opinion former.

For this reason, I can't provide an all-inclusive listing of the components of professionalism. All the characteristics included, however, are those I have heard from more than one person or from one other person with whom I agree. There is no scientific rigor to these observations; they are simply my personal assessments. I'm using the literary device of alliteration to make these professional qualities easier to remember. This is clearly a gimmick, but I'm using it for my own benefit. If you find it distracting, feel free to substitute your own words. That my elements of professionalism all start with the letter "C" means nothing—

but the elaborations on each do mean something. So now, let's embark on the seven "Cs."

The medical professional is *caring*. To the professional, the patient is not "your 11:45" or "the hip replacement" or "the granny with helmet hair." The patient is Mr. Schindler if you are Dr. Doe or Mr. Doe. Occasionally, the caring professional may address a patient by his or her first name, but only if that professional has established a first-name relationship. And then, the professional gets the first name right. I'm Tom, not Thomas or Tommy. If the professional doesn't know my name, especially since it should be on the chart, I wonder if he or she cares.

The professional shows care by attending to little things, by recognizing that what may seem minor in the medical world can be very frightening or intimidating to a patient. Ask yourself what your father would want to hear: "That toe is full of gangrene; it's got to go" or "Your toe is full of poison. The only way we can be sure of saving your leg is to cut off your toe. Other patients who have had this done tell me they were surprised how little the loss of the toe affected their walking. And all of them are still walking—on their own two legs." Which approach is more caring? Which approach would you want used with your loved one? My dad heard both "explanations"—one from each of two providers. I know which one he appreciated.

A second "C" is *comedy*. It is actually a "sense of humor," but that doesn't work with my literary device. People like to laugh. Laughter can provide perspective. Laughter can ease tension. The medical professional should not try to behave like a stand-up comedian, but he or she should make it clear that a little teasing or kidding around is welcome. If the professional can laugh at himself or herself, so much the better. The folks I would most readily recommend are the people who can smile and make me smile. That simple act of human warmth tells me I'm dealing with a healer and not just a mechanic.

The next "C" is *competence*. All medical staff members have the advantage of being considered competent simply because they are in the jobs they have. Competence, however, is not the same as omnipotence. (Lucky for me, because it doesn't start with "C.") The harshest criticisms I've heard about medical staff members relate to a self-perception of omnipotence. "Because she's a doctor (or works for a doctor) she thinks she can do no wrong." "He thinks butter doesn't melt in his mouth." "He acts like he knows everything; even God must go to him for advice."

On the other hand, people appreciate a humble attitude. "As smart as she is, she took time to listen to what I felt about having my knee replaced at such a 'young' age." "He wasn't afraid to admit his mistake, but he made sure I understood what it meant and how he'd try to fix it." With all this, however, I do want my doctor to know what he or she is talking about.

A fourth "C" is *cooperation*. After my accident I saw how important it is for medical staff members to work as a team. And the team is made up of a lot more than physicians. I saw (or was seen by) a raft of M.D.s: trauma specialists, neurologists, physiatrists, orthopedists, internists. All played an important part in my recovery. Yet the people I spent the most time with were the nurses and therapists. These were the people who knew me best, who recognized when I needed a new med and who made sure I got it, who challenged me to try a new therapy routine or to stay with an old routine I couldn't master. They made sure all the doctors knew what was going on with my progress or lack of progress. Because all the staff members worked so well together, because they excelled at cooperation, I got the care I needed. Their cooperative efforts made it possible for me even to write this article less than one year after my traumatic brain injury.

A fifth "C" is *comprehension*. ("Understanding" might be better, but it doesn't fit my pattern.) The professional medical provider tries to understand the patient and doesn't give up until he or she is sure what the patient means. "I don't want to be poked anymore" could mean "I'm tired of waiting for hours for a five-minute test," or it could mean "I'm really afraid of this surgery; I'm afraid I'll die, or end up a vegetable." Comprehension means doing whatever it takes to learn what the patient means or needs and then responding appropriately. People who rave about their doctors say, "They really listen."

The next "C" is *courtesy*. The professional medical provider treats not only patients but also colleagues with courtesy. Courtesy derives from respect. Haughtiness or self-righteousness have no place in professionalism. Professional behavior is courteous behavior. A patient deserves and expects to be treated with dignity—from promptness in appointments to sincere apologies when things don't go right. Similarly, a colleague should know his talents are valued, that he won't be criticized in front of other team members or patients. The last thing I, as a patient, want to hear is criticism from one of my providers about another. Disagreement is fine—that's why we get second opinions—but having to listen to criticism is not welcome. Respect and courtesy are the oil that keeps things running smoothly.

The seventh "C" is *communication*. It is not enough for medical professionals to have knowledge of their field; they also have to share that knowledge. Communicating with their colleagues is usually not much of a challenge; they all speak the same language. Speak that language to a patient, however, and that patient's eyes glaze over. Few things irritate a patient more than spending half a day in the clinic only to leave without having any idea why it is important to come back tomorrow for some "procedure." The medical team may well understand that the patient's "duodenum calcification might anesthetize the prosthesis without intervention, and discomfort might occur without suturing the sinus rhythm of the TBI," but such an "explanation" might as well be in a foreign language as far as the patient is concerned. The terminology leads to nonsense rather than communication. Any hope of the patient's being a partner in his or her own recovery flies right out the window when there is no communication.

So what are the qualities that typify a medical professional? The professional not only knows what he or she is doing, but makes sure patients and colleagues understand it as well. The professional treats both patients and team members the way he or she wants a dearest loved one to be treated. The professional is human, not a robot, who is not afraid to show care and understanding. Listen to your friends and family; they'll tell you what they expect in a professional.

The professionals who cared for me after my accident also cared *about* me. They laughed with me. They knew how to help me and worked together to do it. They understood what I needed. They treated me with respect. Finally, they made sure I understood what I had to do to make a successful recovery. They were both capable *and* kind. They were true professionals.

16

The Role of Reflection in Professionalism Education

Erin A. Egan, M.D., J.D., editor

Most definitions of professionalism or descriptions of competence in professionalism use words like "integrity," "trust," "compassion," "empathy," "altruism," and "honesty."[1] One of the fundamental problems with professionalism education is how to teach such amorphous principles. Clearly, this educating to ensure competency deviates from the traditional educational model of lectures and content testing. Trainees observe this difficulty and are often suspicious of professionalism curricula for that reason. Some even interpret the existence of these curricula as an accusation that they aren't honest, trustworthy, compassionate, or empathetic. However, professionalism education is a process of teaching professionals to recognize optimal manifestations of these traits in professional behavior and encourage active modeling based on that recognition. Reflection is central to that personal exploration of recognition and modeling of desired professional traits.

It is a valid observation that values associated with professionalism such as honesty and integrity cannot be taught in lectures and probably cannot be taught to adults who are genuinely unfamiliar with them. Most, we hope all, students who begin medical school are people of integrity, generally honest and compassionate, capable of empathy, worthy of trust, and trusting of others. The purpose of teaching professionalism is to teach students to expand their experience with these traits and foster them in their professional development. A professionalism curriculum cannot and will not have any effect on psychological outliers who lack a capacity for empathy or honesty, but instead, it targets the normal people who enter medicine. The presumption is that these students have and exemplify these traits, and the focus is on guiding their development.

If professionalism can't be taught the way subjects are traditionally taught in medical school, we need to develop the skills as teachers and learners to expand our modalities. Educators with experience repeatedly emphasize the crucial role of reflection.[2] The reflections included in this book all emphasize the degree to which experience, and the cognitive processing of experience, influence professional development. Using reflection as a primary tool for professionalism education emphasizes experience and reinforces learners' own strengths and perceptions. The focus on analytic introspection of personal experience makes the teaching and learning of professionalism a practical and clinically valuable undertaking.

Reflection is a process that comes naturally to some people, often in the form of writing or journaling. In creating this collection, we solicited reflective pieces and, therefore, most likely ended up with reflections from people predisposed to written reflection. Some medical professionals are not naturally reflective and aren't comfortable with the process. The process of reflecting is a tangible skill that can and should be taught. When the question of how professionalism can be taught arises, the answer is that the skills for professional development can be taught, notably that critical self-reflection can be taught. Ongoing and self-motivated clinical enrichment practices are "forced" on students and residents until they become habitual in the form of journal discussions and discussion of relevant literature on clinical rounds. Trainees suffer consequences for not practicing ongoing patient-centered learning so they will have the desire to continue the practice after training. Similarly, reflection should be actively encouraged and even required until it becomes habitual.

Part of habituating reflection is providing adequate opportunity and outlet for reflection. Journaling is one option that has the advantage of being private and leaving the option to share within the control of the writer. In the training environment, reflection assignments are similar to journaling, but are typically reviewed and are therefore not as private. It is important to create other options such as group reflections on shared experiences for people who aren't comfortable with writing. If a group participates in an activity, particularly a service activity or one that is highly emotionally charged, a subsequent shared reflection can help all members capitalize on positive experiences and process negative ones.

Developing a curriculum that requires reflection is often met with resistance by trainees. Residents in particular question the value of reflection given the medical knowledge requirements and direct patient care obligations they face. The first step to overcoming this resistance is a genuine commitment to the value of reflection by the faculty. Faculty examples of personal reflection, either oral or written, and active participation by faculty members in group reflection experiences are important. Unfortunately, some faculty members are even more resistant to reflection than trainees are. Tacit negative feedback about the value of reflection is particularly destructive when students or residents are already resistant. Therefore, faculty development is a crucial adjunct to implementing any professionalism curriculum, particularly one involving reflection.[3]

Encouraging brief journal entries on a daily basis can encourage regular reflection. Optionally, these can be shared in group environments or used as a basis for written reflection. Finally, involving trainees in developing new curricula and incorporating their input on how they are comfortable incorporating reflection into their own professional development maximizes their acceptance of the process and their comfort level with it.

The collection of reflections in this book represents several areas and styles of reflection both by physicians primarily in training and physicians primarily in practice. The reflections of those early in their professional development illustrate the point that trainees mostly need reinforcement of their own critical analysis and insight applied to significant experiences. List and Krautkramer bring the perspective of preprofessionals, observing professionals with a critical eye to creating a self-definition of professionalism. Jacques, Boyte, and McNeal each look for meaningful insight into formative experiences. Jacques faces a therapeutic interaction with a patient who cannot be cured, and observes that the subsequent relationship is as much for his own benefit as the patient's. The insight that the interaction is mutually beneficial, particularly since this patient was encountered so early in this physician's clinical career, creates a framework for balancing the pain and frustration of caring for such patients with the beauty of providing comfort regardless of cure. The relationship that develops embodies compassion and empathy, and the process of reflection cements those characteristics as valuable and admirable. Boyte struggles with a "difficult" family member, but finds he learns something from her as he forces her down a path toward acknowledging her grief. He is critical of his own behavior ("After all, I had yelled at the mother of a dead girl"), but he ultimately shows compassion and understanding for the woman's pain and the value of her insight. McNeal describes negative role modeling, an unfortunately common experience, but also observes that "Dr. Smith never apologized for his unprofessional behavior." Negative role modeling is particularly important when unprofessional behavior is tolerated, because it undermines our professional assertions that such behavior is intolerable. Reflection helps properly frame the experience despite the lack of insight by the perpetrator, and it promotes the integrity of the trainees in striving to avoid such behavior even when it has no apparent direct consequences.

Several of these reflections are those of educators, either demonstrating their own struggles with teaching professionalism or the experiences of students exposed to structured programs of reflection and professional development. Baernstein examines the common process by which students dismiss scenarios as "unrealistic" when most honest practitioners will admit to experiencing such a scenario at least once. This highlights the challenge of using vicarious experience to teach compassion but still persevering to prepare students to "behave humanely even when they don't feel that way," an expression of integrity. Baernstein also stresses the importance of talking about our less-than-admirable times, acknowledging our imperfections, and using those as strategies for collective improvement. Gibson uses excerpts from actual student reflections to demonstrate the evolution of students' acceptance of the value of reflection and their willingness to analyze how they define and develop professional characteristics. The students demonstrate improved insight into themselves and the professional development process. Doukas and Brennan are experienced educators struggling with the implications of promoting competencies instead of teaching material without specific concern about how behavior is impacted. As they reflect on their own experience with teaching professionalism, they demonstrate both the degree to which promoting professional competence is a function of building on existing skills and traits while critically reflecting on how those traits manifest themselves and the degree to which the instructors grow and develop professionally through their teaching experiences.

The next group of essays represents an important aspect of professional development. Physicians are people, and they sometimes bring their pain, vulnerability, anger, and distaste to professional encounters. Stepien relates the experience of being on the other side of a painful encounter, and leaves unspoken the question of how this encounter will change both parties while acknowledging that it will change them both. Salomon faces a person she has reason to disdain and resent, a person who might pose a physical threat in other circumstances but presents with the vulnerability and dependence common to the state of being a patient. She maintains her professional integrity admirably despite significant inner turmoil. While most of us will not find ourselves in a situation as dramatic as this, where the pain and outrage are so palpable, we will all face personal conflicts with our professional duties. Reflection bears witness to the doctor-person who must acquiesce at times to the doctor-professional. Finally, Ahmed gives insight into potential conflicts with personal beliefs, to which she was fortunately able to find a constructive resolution, a situation that all professionals encounter in some form. Reflecting in this context helps affirm the importance of the principles in conflict on both sides and creates an important resource for others facing similar conflicts. This recognition of important conflicting principles promotes compassion and empathy and allows the professionals to maintain their personal integrity in the face of conflict.

The final reflection is by a patient. The ultimate beneficiaries of the increased emphasis on professionalism in medicine are our patients. Schindler's experience highlights the impact of professionalism. The "seven Cs" are the practical translation of the amorphous traits, mentioned above, that we encourage and foster in professionalism education.

Thus, these essays demonstrate several ways in which reflection can be effective in developing professionalism. They demonstrate a range of possibilities: acknowledging conflicts, analyzing less-than-ideal experiences and behaviors, gaining insight into emotional encounters, striving to maintain human emotion in the face of intense stressors, and treating people humanely despite feelings and inclinations to do otherwise. As professionals, in training or otherwise, reflect in these ways, their emotional experiences promote empathy, their humane behavior in the face of values conflict promotes integrity, their recognition of conflict and attempts to resolve it productively promote trust and trustworthiness, and their acknowledgment of their own shortcomings promotes compassion and empathy. Thus, the reflections here have demonstrated that while professional values cannot be taught in the paradigm of traditional medical education, they can be developed and promoted and, most importantly, encouraged and reinforced. My final observation comes from the experience of reviewing reflections for this collection. Reflection needs to be, for lack of a better word, reflective. It demands some analysis of thoughts and feelings and some insight into behaviors and ways in which behavior can be optimized. Beyond that inherent self-evaluative component, it is important to refrain from qualitative criticism. No reflection is "wrong," and the expressions chosen by the writer and speaker are the best expressions for that individual's experience and should be immune from editing. Sharing of similar experiences, reinforcement of important insights, and empathy and compassion are important feedback when reflections are shared, but the process of reflection needs to be valued for itself and not its product. The process is the educational tool, and the interaction that results from shared reflection magnifies the effect but cannot be allowed to become the educational tool itself.

This collection is designed to encourage reflection through demonstration and to teach professionalism through shared experience with professional growth. It is intended to show how values like empathy, integrity, honesty, altruism, compassion, and trust can be taught or, more accurately, promoted and nurtured. The readers we hope to reach are professionals, professional students (medical students and residents), and professional educators. Professionalism is an important dynamic entity to all these groups, one that needs to evolve to reflect the issues professionals must face. Reflection keeps the process fresh and dynamic, current to the needs of the professionals. Without a prominent focus on experience and reflection, the "field" of professionalism runs the risk of stagnating. Without continuous affirmation of the variability of clinical encounters and professional responses to those encounters, professionalism will become narrow and outdated. Reflection respects our creativity, our identity, and our commitment to self-improvement in changing and growing as professionals.

NOTES

1. For some commonly referred to descriptions of professionalism as a competency, see ABIM Foundation, ACP-ASIM Foundation, and European Feder-

ation of Internal Medicine, "Medical Professionalism in the New Millennium, a Physician Charter," *Annals of Internal Medicine* 2002; 136: 243–46 (available at www.abimfoundation.org/pdf/charter.pdf); ACGME Outcomes Project, "Competencies, Professionalism" (available atwww.acgme.org/outcome/comp/compFull.asp#5).

2. For an example of articles discussing the importance of reflection in professional development, see (please note this is an incomplete list of articles on the issue) R. M. Epstein and E. M. Hundert, "Defining and assessing professional competence," *Journal of the American Medical Association* 287(2): 226–35, 9 January 2002; J. J. Fins et al., "Reflective practice and palliative care education: A clerkship responds to the informal and hidden curricula," *Academic Medicine* 78(3): 307–12, March 2003; R. M. Epstein, "Mindful practice," *Journal of the American Medical Association* 282(9): 833–39, 1 September 1999.

3. For example, Rachel Remen, of UCSF School of Medicine and author of *Kitchen Table Wisdom*, has developed a course focusing on reflection called the Healer's Art, taught at many medical schools. Part of the course involves training the moderators of the reflection groups on effective practices in group reflection and creating a productive group dynamic.

Index

Contributors

EDITORS

Erin A. Egan, M.D., J.D., is an assistant professor at the Neiswanger Institute for Bioethics and Health Policy, and in the Division of General Internal Medicine at Loyola University Medical Center.

Patricia M. Surdyk, Ph.D., is executive director for the Institutional Review Committee of the Accreditation Council for Graduate Medical Education (ACGME).

INVITED ESSAYISTS

Gwen L. Nichols, M.D., is the director of the Hematologic Malignancies Program at Columbia University College of Physicians and Surgeons and an associate attending physician in hematology and oncology.

Alison S. Clay, M.D., is a clinical associate in critical care medicine in the Department of Surgery at Duke University Medical Center.

Norma E. Wagoner, Ph.D., retired in June 2002 after twenty-eight years as a student dean in three medical schools. The last fourteen years she served as dean of students and deputy dean for education strategy, Pritzker School of Medicine, The University of Chicago, where she was awarded the University's Gold Key for distinguished service.

CONTRIBUTORS

Mona Ahmed is a third-year medical student at Loyola University Stritch School of Medicine.

Amy Baernstein, M.D., is assistant professor of medicine at the University of Washington School of Medicine and an attending physician in the Emergency Trauma Center at Harborview Medical Center.

W. Richard Boyte, M.D., is associate professor of pediatrics in the Department of Pediatrics at the University of Mississippi School of Medicine.

Mark G. Brennan is head of division of clinical education at Kent Institute of Medicine & Health Sciences, University of Kent, Canterbury, UK.

David J. Doukas, M.D., is the William Ray Moore Endowed Chair of Family Medicine and Medical Humanism, and Chief, Division of Medical Humanism and Ethics at the University of Louisville.

Justin M. List is a second-year medical student at Loyola University Stritch School of Medicine and a former fellow in the Ethics Group of the American Medical Association.

Andrew P. Jacques is an emergency medicine resident at Akron General Medical Center in Akron, Ohio, and a 2005 graduate of Wright State University School of Medicine.

Christian J. Krautkramer is a senior research assistant in the Ethics Group of the American Medical Association.

Denise D. Gibson, Ph.D., is assistant dean, academic support and associate professor, clinical psychiatry at the University of Cincinnati College of Medicine.

Sandra McNeal is a fourth-year medical student at the University of Illinois, Chicago.

Bonnie Salomon, M.D., is an emergency physician at Lake Forest Hospital and teaches medical ethics at Lake Forest College.

Thomas Schindler has visited, worked in, and been admitted to a variety of health care facilities in the Chicago area over the past forty years. In February 2005, he was in a serious traffic accident that required extended treatment for a traumatic brain injury. He works in an administrative office position with no health care involvement.

Kathy Stepien, M.A., P.T., is a medical student at the University of Washington School of Medicine. She resides in Seattle with her husband, Jim, and their son, Will.